CW00351074

# SOUNDS LIKE
## Skipper

# Kerena Marchant

## SOUNDS LIKE
# Skipper

**The story of Kerena Marchant
and her hearing dog Skipper**

Hodder & Stoughton

LONDON SYDNEY AUCKLAND TORONTO

*British Library Cataloguing in Publication Data*

Marchant, Kerena
  Sounds like Skipper : the story of
  Kerena Marchant and her hearing dog,
  Skipper.
  1. Deaf—Psychology
  I. Title
  362.4'2'0924      HV2395

  ISBN 0-340-39154-5

# Contents

Deafness is a frustrating world of silence, where lips either move silently or voices can be sometimes heard as a meaningless mumble. It is like a high wall, and a deaf person can so easily be isolated on one side whilst hearing people can live unaware of the deaf on the other side of that wall. But it is a wall that can be crossed if the will and the strength are there.

This book is dedicated to my family, friends – canine and human – teachers and colleagues who have helped me.

# Illustrations

CREDITS

| | |
|---|---|
| 1 *Daily Telegraph* | 2 Mike Binns |
| 3 Colin Ramsey | 4 BBC Enterprises |
| 5 *Dumfries & Galloway Standard* | |

# 1

# Playground Whispers

It was a warm July evening and I was sitting in the ruins of Aberystwyth castle where over two thousand townsfolk and holiday-makers had gathered to sing their Songs of Praise. A small boy called Sam in a group of school-children held my attention, for, like me, he was deaf. Anxious that he should be seen and see everything, his proud school-teachers had pushed him to the front of the congregation, several rows in front of his school-friends, teachers and parents. Frustrated, and wondering what on earth was happening, he decided to face the congregation so that he could see and try to understand exactly what was going on. There were frantic efforts to make him face the right way, and nobody seemed to understand his stubborn decision to face the wrong way, except myself.

The situation suddenly made me feel very sad as I began to think of the many problems that this little boy would have to overcome and the countless misunderstandings he would be subjected to. As I looked at his parents, I wondered if their happy smiles masked the strain that they faced, bringing up a deaf child. Sam had gone deaf after an attack of meningitis when he was very young. Despite the fact that deafness is a very common side-effect of meningitis, neither his doctors nor his parents discovered that he was deaf until a year after his illness.

How incredible! many people might think, but deafness in children is something that can be discovered very late. Psychologists have wrestled to give a credible

9

explanation for this, and their answer is a simple one. A bright child who goes deaf within the first two years or so of its life will "tune in" to its family. The child will subconsciously learn to understand their lip-patterns, their movements, their habits, and thus assimilate its routine.

Even today I've noticed that the better I get to know people the easier it is to understand them. Often, I even jump the gun with those I know well and say, "All right, let's do that," before they have even had a chance to speak. Most of my friends laugh at this and say I'm psychic, but they forget that speech is only a small part of communication – the facial expressions, the gestures they use and the vibes they project when they speak, feelings of happiness, anger or frustration, and lip-patterns all say as much or more than speech.

Understanding is one problem, communicating another. "Slow to learn to talk" on a record sheet will explain away the child's bad speech or lack of it, and conscientious hearing parents like mine will go to endless effort to improve the child's speech. Laziness, disobedience or lack of concentration are produced as reasons for why the child refuses to respond when its back is turned. Many times I remember being dragged away from playing with my dolls or exploring a corner of our flat and being smacked. I now suppose that someone must have been calling me and, because I didn't come, I was punished for disobedience.

Deafness is never thought of – it is not a disability that can be seen. A blind child may be seen to have unfocused eyes or to grope around; a deaf child is a copycat who learns to compensate for its disability at an early age.

I remember my grandfather pointing to a deer in Richmond Park. "You see that deer that has just run away, whilst the others keep grazing, Kerena? That deer is deaf. How do I know? It's more alert than the others, see. They can graze lazily on, relying on their ears. That one uses its eyes and its nose. A blind or a lame deer couldn't survive. But a deaf deer can, if it is bright and uses every sense it has got."

Deafness in a child is often discovered when the child leaves its family environment and goes to school or playgroup and encounters strange people. My own deafness was not discovered until I started at a small private primary school in Kensington at the age of five. The family traumas of my early years were partly to blame for this. My parents separated and my father, an Iranian, stayed in his own country, leaving my mother to bring me up in England without any support from him whatsoever. My mother, being a resourceful woman, overcame these problems by doing as many jobs as she could cram into twenty-four hours. She was a millionaire's secretary, doctor's receptionist and university student's thesis-typist all at the same time.

This meant that I was mostly looked after by my grandparents, who had to keep a close eye on me in case my father attempted to snatch me and take me back to Iran with him, as he had attempted to do before mum had me made a ward of court. British justice had given mum custody of me; but she and my grandparents were very aware that if my father were to succeed in getting me to Iran, they would never see me again, so they took no chances. I went everywhere with my grandparents or my mother. I was not allowed to wander off and play with other children in the park, or talk to any strangers. We moved to a new area and contact with several family friends was broken, in case my father learned where we were. Thus mine was a small, enclosed world of three people – my grandparents and my mother.

The day I started primary school was a disaster. My comfortable world of three had suddenly expanded into a large group of strange children and teachers who did not know me. I did not know how to behave with them and even to this day I remember my early days at primary school as a hazy nightmare.

I had only been there a few weeks when the head teacher called my mother to the school. The teacher explained that all I did in free-expression classes was to sit cross-legged and do nothing. (Mother resisted the temptation to tell her that this was a form of free expression!) The teacher's simple explanation for my behaviour and lack of communication was that I was backward – but mum did not agree with that theory! However, she did take the teacher's observation seriously and discussed the problem with the family doctor, who subsequently discovered that I was deaf.

This discovery shocked the family. Why hadn't they realised? When did I go deaf? The doctors diagnosed my deafness as profound congenital nerve-deafness, but were unable to say exactly what had brought it about. There are a number of explanations, but this is the most feasible. When I was still quite young, I had a very severe illness, and we think that I was treated with sulphonamide, a drug which has been known to cause deafness in some people, and mum is almost sure that is what happened.

In the early sixties there were no high-powered hearing-aids available to children. Those that were lacked the correct powers of amplification needed to reach the very little residual hearing I had and were unable to work like a graphic equaliser and amplify middle frequencies. All they did was make the few very high or very low sounds that I could hear chronically loud, causing extreme pain and possible damage to my ears. The high-powered Phonac hearing-aids I have today are capable of amplifying certain sounds more than others, and are more powerful than the aids available when I was young. When I was a child, sound was an infrequent whisper, like the sound of the sea in a shell, far away in another world, but comforting. I loved play-time at school, when, if I concentrated hard enough, the whispers of children shouting penetrated my silence. Today what I hear is similar to what somebody must hear when they swim under water: a faint garble, with the odd word or sound being clear if it is familiar.

As there is no medical cure for nerve-deafness and the hearing-aids of my childhood were inadequate, the doctor prescribed a dog to keep me company. How perceptive that doctor was! It is easy for a deaf child to communicate with a dog, which only speaks with doggy gestures. As we lived in a flat in Shepherd's Bush, it was decided that a small dog was essential and, after a long search, we eventually acquired Sam, a mischievous Jack Russell puppy from the Pound Hill Kennels in Crawley. Sam became my childhood playmate in countless games together. I'd chase Sam around the dining-room table until I caught his tail, then he'd chase me until I caught his paw. He never minded being dressed up in dolls' clothes or being woken up at night to raid the fridge. At a time when I was confused and struggling to come to terms with what was going on around me, Sam's uncomplicated company was a welcome escape. And, even to this day, when I need to relax it is always the company of animals that I seek.

Most days, before I started going to school, gran and I would go out somewhere, and each outing was a lesson. "Bu-airs," she'd say, and point to the bears in the London Zoo and I'd try and copy her. When I eventually got it right, she gave me something to throw to the bears, who did not have "No feeding" notices outside their cages in those days! "Bu-loo," she'd say when she was doing a blue-wash at home. The reward for getting that right was a sweet or a game. Fortunately, she was a determined, patient person, blessed with a sense of humour and backed by my mother and my grandfather when they returned from work in the evening, and my step-father, Peter, when he came into our lives.

I can never understand, when I look back on those early days, why I never knew that I was deaf.

I don't know when I came to terms with my deafness, as it was a gradual process, which to a certain extent is still going on today! I cannot even remember the exact moment when I knew that I *was* deaf – when I realised that the lips that moved silently should make a noise; that the everyday movements around me were accompanied by noise. Silent lips made meaningful patterns, for I had acquired a deaf child's inherent ability to read lips and face-patterns, and to "feel" what mood the speaker was in. Things made lots of different vibrations – my toy flute and drum; the piano; the TV and the car. Being deaf was as natural as being hearing until I gradually realised that I communicated differently and was regarded as being different by some people.

In the early sixties the only way to improve a child's speech was by painstaking efforts. Words were mouthed clearly in separate syllables, or if a child could read, written down phonetically. A deaf child was encouraged to touch the speaker's mouth or throat to feel the sounds, to watch tongue and teeth positions and, if possible, copy them. My family's efforts at home were supplemented by those of a speech-therapist. Today, teaching a deaf child to speak is made easier by the use of computers. A word is spoken into a computer and a pattern is made on the screen. The deaf child tries to copy the pattern when he repeats the word.

My family, however, treated me as a normal child and never let my deafness be an excuse for anything. I remember my mother teaching me to wash my hair and telling me that I could tell when I had got all the soap out of my hair by running my fingers through my hair and hearing the squeak. "Can't hear it!" I wailed, throwing one of my numerous childhood tantrums. "You don't have to hear it," said Peter, my calm stepfather, who had added an air of family stability to my life when I was eight. "Run your fingers through your hair and see if it tickles. If it does, you've got the soap out."

If my parents treated me as a normal child who just happened to be deaf, my primary-school teachers did not. I was made to sit on my own away from the other children. If I tried to sit with them, I was dragged back to my solitary desk in a corner at the front, unless it was singing or music, when I was given a recorder and sent to a room on my own to play it. My books were different to the other children's and did not look as important. Because of the teachers' treatment, I was the odd one out – different. It took me a long time to make a friend, but everything changed when Amanda Bull, the daughter of an Ear, Nose and Throat consultant, decided that I was to be her friend. Instead of playing on my own, I played with the other kids who were marvellous! If we played Chinese whispers, a game where a message is whispered round a circle, the kids would shut their eyes while someone mouthed the message to me. If I said something wrong or mispronounced something, Amanda would patiently help me to understand or to pronounce it correctly, supplementing my family's efforts at home. If I was by now aware that I was missing out on a thing called noise, I was at least ceasing to feel different.

Often today someone working with the deaf, or even deaf people themselves, say, "But you're not really deaf – you talk and understand me so well," – intended compliments which only succeed in irritating me, because learning to speak well was a hard slog and involved a lot of dedication from my family, teachers and school-friends. Life was not a bed of roses in a normal school, but it did mean that I was always surrounded by hearing people who constantly corrected my speech and commented on my voice. Often somebody would say something like, "It's not wharrr, it's wh-at. Look at me, wha-AT. It's a hard sound from the back of the throat followed by a "t", tongue behind the front teeth." Or, "Your voice is boring and flat. I'll write out a sentence on a musical scale for you and underline the words you must pronounce more, and you must try and say words as you feel them. If you're happy, emphasise happy words." These remarks started as early as I can recall, with my grandparents and mother at home. I'd often get so frustrated because I couldn't have my pudding or something nice as I couldn't say the word for it, and had to learn how to say it first. This has continued up to the present day, with my colleagues correcting my mispronunciations at work.

Learning the hard way like this was humiliating at times. My grandmother would send me into a shop with the right money and point to what she wanted and I had to ask for it. Sometimes the shop assistants would not understand and give me the wrong thing, but more and more often they did understand and my confidence grew.

When the eleven-plus examinations came up, my parents were summoned to the school and told I had no chance of ever passing them; that I was a dim, badly behaved, backward child who would certainly never be able to go to a grammar school and would have to go to a special school, possibly one for the deaf, if I was bright enough for that. This news came as a great shock to my parents who had never been led to believe that this was the case from my school reports. Both were against sending me to a school for the deaf as they felt that since one day I would have to work in the hearing world, the sooner I learnt to cope in it the better. They were also anxious that I continue to be surrounded by hearing children who would correct my speech. As I was already integrating well with the children at school and beginning to overcome my problems for myself, they thought it would be a shame to stop my progress.

However, many people who work with the deaf and many deaf people themselves might think that my parents made the wrong decision, and I do agree that the sink-or-swim situation a deaf child is faced with in a normal school is one that many deaf kids can't always cope with. But, to me it was a challenge. Even if I didn't realise it at the time, going through the trauma, heartbreak, humiliation and happiness of a normal education equipped me for university and my present job in the tough world of broadcasting. Not everybody is understanding about my deafness and wants to help; many people want to help but don't know how to. Frequently, a new relationship requires at first an eighty per cent effort on my part, and this is something that I have, over the years, taught myself to handle.

It was obvious that I would have to go to a school where there were small classes, so a large London comprehensive was out. Deep down my parents knew that I was bright, even if my teachers and psychologists at the hospital disagreed with them. Eventually, they decided to send me to Battle Abbey, a fee-paying boarding school in Sussex. They had faith in me, and were prepared to work long hours and go without so much in order to give me a chance. It was a great sacrifice and they were unsure if they had made the right decision. I know that going to a school for the deaf would have been cheaper for them and have demanded less effort on my part, for less would have been expected of me. At Battle I had to do everything, and there were no concessions.

I'll never forget my first week at Battle! I was left at this boarding school, surrounded by unknown people – terrified and homesick. As I was unsure of myself, I made no attempts to find friends. Then, a week later, when I had settled down, I found out why no one had tried to make friends with me! "We thought you were foreign and didn't speak much English, because you don't speak much and when you do your speech is peculiar." But when the others found out that I was deaf, they couldn't have been more supportive. In every lesson, there was always someone ready to take notes for me or to explain what went on afterwards. Teachers were generally good about not facing the blackboard, but when they did, a chorus of "Don't face the board; Kerena can't lip-read you!" was always uttered by the rest of the class.

Miss Mumford, the history teacher, was wonderful. She not only took care to write down all the facts on the blackboard, she even sat her class in a semicircle and made them put up their hands when they wanted to talk, so that I could follow a discussion. Miss Scott, my form teacher, Mrs Gould, the RE teacher and Miss Fentumn, the English teacher, all gave me extra lessons to help improve my grammar and spelling; and Miss Parker, the head teacher, was quick to correct my speech and help my pronunciation, but if I learnt a lot from my teachers, I learnt just as much from my friends.

Every term a class had to take assembly and people

would be selected to read. I was never chosen and eventually, I asked my best friend, Angie, why this was. "Well, I think you're doing three things wrong. Firstly, you're not able to judge how loud you're speaking, and when you tried to read, we couldn't hear you at the back. Secondly, you get nervous and your voice goes squeaky, and, thirdly, your voice is flat and boring. But don't worry, I'll help." I was well aware that there were different notes on a piano by vibration and could read music, so Angie wrote down a sentence on a music scale, with all the words on different lines, and some were in capitals.

"What you must do," explained the thirteen-year-old Angie, "is to go up and down when you speak and put more feeling into the words in capitals. Feel happy about saying them." For a month we practised that. Then came the next stage. "You go on the platform and I'll stand at the back of the hall; if you start squeaking, I'll tell you by raising my hand, and if I can't hear you, I'll put my hand behind my ear. OK?" We practised this for a few weeks, and when the form teacher auditioned us for reading in assembly, I was chosen. "Well done," said Angie, who should have taken the credit. "Don't worry about doing it, because I'll stand at the back." She did and I was fine.

Assembly was one hurdle; school plays were another. I wanted a good speaking part, but never got one. But once I'd done assembly, I was confident that I could do a play.

"No problem," said Angie, "but you'll have to learn about accents and learn how to talk with one." Angie, a natural actress herself, began to talk in different accents. I noticed her lips making different patterns. She then wrote down some words of a poem we had been doing in drama to show the accent. "TaeNooo-a-way, taeNoo-a-way! The King's daughter aee Nooraway tis th-aa maaee bring her hame." We practised along these lines with much amusement for the rest of the term, and I became very aware of accents. What amazed me later when I met other deaf people, was that they all spoke with strong regional accents, most probably learnt from regional lip-patterns!

Next term I auditioned for a part in Christopher Fry's *Boy With A Cart*, and got one of the main parts: a grumpy old man called Tawm. "I'll teach you to do the West-Country accent," Angie volunteered, writing down my lines phonetically and patiently listening to them again and again. But accents were not my only problem. Like all comedy roles, playing Tawm demanded perfect timing. I had to say my lines on time and couldn't miss a cue. "Don't worry," said the rest of the cast, "we'll always give you visual cues as well, and if something goes wrong, we'll ad-lib until we get to your next cue." This plan worked very well in *Boy With A Cart* and all the other plays I acted in at Battle. People scratched their heads, got handkerchieves out of their pockets, and nobody in the audience ever guessed these were my cues, not just part of the show.

These plays gave me enormous self-confidence, because I had to do the same as everybody else; no allowances were made for me. I got the parts because I auditioned and earned them, just the same as everybody else, and began to realise that if I could do this on these terms, I could do most things. Admittedly, I worked harder than the rest of the cast, for I had to learn all my lines before the first rehearsal so that I could look at people to understand what they were saying and keep an eye out for my visual cues; I had to learn to pronounce difficult words correctly as well as to speak with an accent – and to work out how to put various emotions into words. But it was worthwhile, because my speech got better and better as my confidence grew.

On the sports field, it was much the same as in class.

"It's not fair!" I once complained to the games teacher, "I should get a twenty-yard start because I can't hear the gun. When you start the race with your hand, I win; when you start it with a word or a gun, I lose."

At the time her response seemed very unsympathetic, though it was hammering home a familiar lesson. "You'll have to run faster, then. Life isn't fair, and if you think that you will be given chances later on, you're very wrong."

I learnt to run a little faster!

I wanted to succeed in life for a number of reasons: to reward my parents, teachers and friends for their hard work and patience with me and to prove that any handicap can be overcome if there's a way and a will – especially now there are countless environmental aids to help equalise the balance between disabled people and everybody else. I see no reason why disabled people should not have normal ambitions and fight on an equal footing to achieve them or to fail, just as other people do. It simply takes a little bit of confidence, and people to help that confidence grow, and a lot more effort – but disabled people often have more incentive to succeed!

Looking at the small boy in Aberystwyth, desperately trying to fathom out what everybody else was doing standing around the castle, made me realise how far I had come from the frightened, unsure primary-school child to the more confident BBC researcher.

Suddenly, I felt a gentle paw urgently tapping my knee and saw Skipper, my Hearing Dog, staring at me with a sense of purpose. "What is it?" I asked. With an important air about him, the little Jack Russell turned and led me to the stage manager, who had called him and told him to go and get me. I had Skipper, my ears, my environmental aid that I could take anywhere, to thank for enabling me to do my job as well as my hearing colleagues and for giving me a large amount of confidence.

# 2

# Sitting On The Stairs

I was anxiously waiting on the stairs leading up to my flat, with the front-door open. Thankfully, it was spring, so it wasn't too cold. I have waited many times for the gas or electricity man to call in mid-winter, freezing cold, with the door open wide. Sitting on the hall stairs with the door open isn't the usual way to await the arrival of a caller, but when you're deaf and can't hear a doorbell, you don't have much choice. Flashing-light doorbells are available, but some are not easy to see in bright daylight, and flashing lights that anyone in the street can also see going on and off are not very good for security!

For the past year I had been living in my own flat – independent, with a mortgage – but very cut off. Often, friends would say, "I called, but you were out," when I knew that I'd been in, but had not heard the doorbell. On the whole, friends were very good at arriving at a pre-arranged time, but other callers weren't. "We can't make appointments, or even let you know roughly when we'll arrive," seems to be the motto of British Telecom, the electricity, the gas-board and delivery men. Explanations about how you are deaf and can't hear the doorbell, and that you can't really ask a friend to take a morning off work to be there, fall on "deaf ears".

Today I was waiting for someone very special: Gillian Lacey, the placement counsellor from Hearing Dogs for the Deaf. Gillian, of course, understood my problem and had agreed to call between four and five o'clock. I was very nervous because she was coming to see if I really needed a Hearing Dog and if I was suitable to own one, since my flat was very small for a dog to live in. I had read about Hearing Dogs for the Deaf on *No Need to Shout*, a magazine for the hearing-impaired on Ceefax, the BBC's Teletext service. "Hearing Dogs are similar to Guide Dogs for the Blind," I read. "They alert their deaf owners when everyday noises that hearing people take for granted sound off: doorbells, phones, a knock at the door, a baby crying, burglars and fire-alarms – as well as providing friendship." Living on my own, I needed that help, and at work, too.

I was working then as a subtitler for the deaf and hard-of-hearing in Ceefax on a number of popular television series from a script and video-cassette of the programmes. As I often worked late shifts and was in the office on my own a lot, fire-alarms were a great worry, especially as I had missed two fire practices!

I had taught myself to use a telephone by attaching a specific vibrating microphone onto a specially amplified telephone. With powerful hearing-aids and intense concentration, I could hear a fraction of sound and supplement that with vibrations from the microphone. Different sounds make different vibrations and you can help yourself by angling the phone conversation to get a distinctive vibration back. So when, say, an engineer rang up, I'd guess that he was calling to let me know the subtitles had broken down, so I would ask what was wrong, and he'd have to say, "the film" or, "the disc", which are words that feel entirely different.

There is also a special phone for the deaf in the office called a Vistel, which is a keyboard with a small visual-display unit. Two people, both with Vistels, can hold a telephone conversation by typing messages which are displayed on the receiving Vistel.

Whilst using a phone was not easy, but not impossible, telling when it rang was! I had a handset with a flashing light, but when I was busy subtitling – something which requires immense concentration if you are deaf – I would never notice it flash. I once had a phone with a flashing light at home, but it broke down and British Telecom seemed unable to find me another. However, I got round this problem to a certain extent at home by placing the phone on the sofa. That way, if I was sitting on the sofa, I could feel it vibrate when the phone rang.

There is no such thing as a burglar-alarm for deaf people, as they are all audio. In fact, burglar-alarms tell everybody else except the deaf householder that there is a burglar on the premises. When I thought about it, it made me feel very vulnerable, as well as cut off.

A Hearing Dog would solve so many of these problems and give me the friendship and protection I needed, living on my own. I would be really independent. However, I did have worries – would the BBC allow a dog to come to work? I thought they might, especially as it was otherwise going to cost £16,000 to wire up our temporary office with a flashing light fire-alarm. A permanent office in the BBC is a myth. Every so often, for some reason, everyone seems to play musical offices and move to a new base – and I could see that moving a flashing-light fire-alarm was not going to be popular.

My real misgivings were about myself as a potential owner. I'd always loved animals and had owned that mischievous Jack Russell called Sam as a child, but I was living in London now in a small flat. I knew a dog would not suffer, living with me, because I love walking, and there were so many parks and open spaces near. But what would the lady from Hearing Dogs think?

Meanwhile, it was six o'clock and she was an hour late. Perhaps I'd misheard and got the wrong day? But one of my colleagues at work had taken the message, and written it down. I was about to embark on one of my minor panics when the door opened. "Hello, I'm Gillian from Hearing Dogs," said an attractive, well-dressed girl of about my age, who spoke very slowly and clearly. "I'm really sorry that I'm so late, but I got held up with an old lady who wouldn't let me get away. I guessed you'd be waiting like this." For once, the long wait didn't matter. The apology was so completely understanding.

"Do you want me to sign, or can you understand me all right?" Gillian asked. As Gillian was speaking so clearly, I didn't need to resort to sign language. It is something I

23

use as a last resort, when I'm tired. Usually, hearing people who know how to sign can't wait to sign at me, so someone who asked first made a welcome change.

"Would you like a cup of coffee?" I asked suddenly, remembering my manners.

"Oh, yes please," replied Gillian, "but first I'd like a bowl of water for my dog."

"Why not bring your dog up?" I suggested, pleased at the prospect of some doggy company.

Gillian disappeared and returned with a rather elegant-looking mongrel. "Her name is Ge-mma," she mouthed clearly, "and she is one of our demonstration dogs." Gemma looked angelically up at me as if to say, I'm sure you would like to have me, but I'm not on offer!

Over coffee and cakes Gillian explained that she had received a copy of my audiogram (hearing test) from the hospital and that I was definitely deaf enough to qualify for a Hearing Dog. She agreed that unless I could take the dog to work, where it was needed, it would be rather unkind to have a dog. But the smallness of my flat didn't seem to bother her. "You'd have to have a small dog," was her only comment. I explained that if I had a small dog I wanted one that was full of energy so I could take it for walks. I didn't want a lap-dog, and I showed Gillian a photo of Sam, who had recently died.

"I don't see any problem in finding a Jack Russell or terrier-type dog," she replied cheerfully. "We always try and get our dogs from the National Canine Defence League kennels and they get plenty of Jack Russells and terriers there."

"So when do you think I will have a dog?" I asked, encouraged by Gillian's enthusiasm.

"Well, first the committee have to approve your case, then we put you on our waiting list and start to keep an eye out for the sort of dog you want. When we find him, it will take a further three to four months to train him. Do you think the chances of you being able to take the dog to work are good?" Gillian asked.

I explained that the request was somewhere in the BBC bureaucracy and that if it hadn't put the bureaucracy out of joint, I should know the result of my request quite soon. At first people in the BBC had thought that a Hearing Dog was a joke, but by the time I'd got the support of the BBC doctor, the personnel officer, as well as the Ceefax management, they began to see the advantages for the Corporation as well as for me.

Gillian and I talked for a while about why I wanted a dog and what I hoped it would do for me. She was also interested to learn about my education, hobbies and ambitions. I explained that whilst I enjoyed subtitling and felt that it was a worthwhile job because of the enjoyment that subtitles gave to so many hearing-impaired people, I felt that I was enclosed in a deaf world and would like to work in a normal production area of the BBC, especially in Religious Programmes as I had a degree in theology.

Eventually, Gillian felt that it was time to leave, though Gemma could have sat contentedly beside the fire for a lot longer. "I'll write to you as soon as the committee comes to a decision," Gillian promised. "And let me know how you get on with the BBC, and if I can help out there." I promised to let her know the day I heard the result of my request and assured her that I could handle the BBC myself.

Every day I anxiously scanned the mail at home and at work, hoping that Hearing Dogs and the BBC would write and say that I could have a dog and take it to work. I tried not to, but I began to build up a picture of the dog in my mind. He was little, shaggy, with legs too small for his body, piebald with bright eyes and a cheeky grin. I even began to go for regular walks in the park, imagining what it would be like to be a dog-owner again. "Don't count your chickens before they've hatched," I kept telling myself.

It was not long before I was asked to go and see the BBC doctor. This made me quite optimistic as he had always been very understanding. When I had applied for a BBC disabled parking-ticket, so I would not have to walk home late at night and could park near the security guards, he was very supportive. He understood a deaf person's fear of walking anywhere alone at night. It really is terrifying

— you can't hear and you can't see and all the time you feel that this is the night you'll be attacked.

The doctor listened with interest as I outlined all the advantages of bringing a dog to the BBC and then asked if many deaf people took their dogs to work. I had been dreading this question. I had to explain that Hearing Dogs was a new scheme and not only would I be one of the first people to own a dog, I would certainly be the first to take their dog to work.

I left the doctor feeling optimistic, however. He hadn't promised anything, but he sounded as if he might be on my side. At long last it was agreed that I could take the dog to work, providing I gave the animal sufficient exercise, and did not take it in the restaurants. That seemed fair enough, and I was thrilled.

Now that it was confirmed that I could take the dog to work, some of my colleagues in Subtitling had a few questions for me. "What are we going to do when deafie dog answers the phone?" asked Sharon, imagining a frantic race between woman and dog to be first to the handset. "Do I have to warn all my friends that if a dog answers, he's barking for you?" I explained that the dog would be trained to tell me when the phone rang by coming up to me, touching me with his paw and leading me to the phone, but he would certainly not answer it! I was quite capable of answering the phone myself, all I couldn't do was hear it ring!

There was also much discussion over what breed "deafie dog" would be. Most people visualised a Labrador or an Alsatian — probably because they are most often used as Guide Dogs for the Blind. But as Hearing Dogs are selected from National Canine Defence League dog-homes, I knew the chances were he would be a mongrel and still hoped he would be a Jack Russell or some ridiculous-looking creature. What he looked like didn't matter, it was what he would be and the vast effect I knew he would have on my life that I thought about.

All the same, I still rushed to open my post, hoping that the photo Gillian had promised to send me of my dog would hurry up and arrive.

# 3

## Enter Skipper

At last, about a month after the BBC had approved the idea of my having a Hearing Dog, the long-awaited letter from Gillian arrived. I could barely open it for excitement, and there inside was a picture of a cheeky-looking Jack Russell, just the kind of dog I would have chosen myself. He was even broken-coated, like my Sam. His tail was unusually long for a Jack Russell, until it occurred to me that he just hadn't had it docked. His ears were brown, and his back black, with a big white spot in the middle – a real hotch-potch, a real Heinz 57! He looked ever so self-confident, standing there, seeming to say, Oh! I wonder why my photo's being taken. He was just the dog for me.

Eventually, I tore myself away from the photo, and read Gillian's letter. The little dog, she wrote, had no name. He was discovered by the police, wandering the back-streets of Stow-on-the-Wold, and taken to the National Canine Defence League kennel. It would be *my* dog that had a police record, I thought! Later on, a few weeks after he had come to live with me, I discovered some of the ways in which he had survived in the back-streets. One day in the park, he actually caught a duck. There was a frantic fight, with fur and feathers flying, before I managed to wrestle the duck away from a fast-moving dog. Chinese take-aways also had a vast attraction for him. If ever he smelt the remains of a Chinese meal in a bin, or when we walked past a Chinese restaurant, he'd stop and sit there, licking his lips and drooling. Thankfully, these bad habits disappeared after six months with me, when he learnt that he could take food for granted, and that he no longer had to fend for himself.

Back to Gillian's letter. It was very important, she wrote, that the little dog should be named as quickly as possible, so that he could be trained to respond to the name I chose. Stella Binns, one of the people who had sponsored Skipper, had suggested three names for him: Skipper, Skippy or Mickey. As there was a certain air of authority about him in the photo, I decided he was a Skipper, and was pleased to discover later that I couldn't have chosen a better name, because Skipper was the name of Stella's dog, who had died.

I was so anxious to let Hearing Dogs know my dog was no longer nameless, that I rushed into my car, rushed to work, and found someone to help me make the phone call. I was so excited, I could hardly speak. Tony Blunt, the training officer, answered the phone, and I explained that I had decided to call the dog Skipper. He too was pleased and said that this was the name he had secretly been calling him.

Now that Skipper had been safely named to everyone's satisfaction, I turned my attention again to Gillian's letter, which I had only skimmed first time through in my rush to name the dog. She was inviting me to attend an open day at the Training Centre, so that I could meet Skipper before he came to live with me and also have a chance to speak to other owners, sponsors, and dogs. I couldn't wait for that day to come, the day when I would meet the dog who was going to change my life.

Wherever I went, I carried a photograph of Skipper. I must have shown it to everyone, at least five times. People were very polite, but I saw a lot of them looking rather surprised to find that Skipper was a funny-looking small mongrel, not an Alsatian or Labrador, as they had imagined he would be.

"Is this thing going to protect you?" David, the Teletext Manager, asked, staring at the photo. "I thought you were getting a Great Dane, or something which could really protect you at night!" I explained to

David that an Alsatian or Great Dane was all very well but in a small office he would not be very comfortable. All the same, there was an air of authority as well in Skipper that inspired me to have confidence in him. Even at that early stage I knew that whatever happened he would look after me when he came.

Alison from *No Need to Shout,* the Teletext magazine for the deaf and hard-of-hearing, offered to come to the open day with me. She thought it would be a good story for the magazine and her presence would give me some moral support. When it came to the point, I found I was actually quite nervous about meeting Skipper for the first time, so I was pleased to have her company on the drive to Oxford.

I arranged to meet Alison in Ealing and arrived at our rendezvous an hour early in my excitement. As luck would have it, it poured with rain while I was waiting, and by the time Alison arrived I was very bedraggled. "Have you been waiting long?" she asked, noticing my very wet appearance.

"Oh no!" I lied. "I just had a long walk from the station," and then suddenly realised that the station was just opposite. Alison was too polite to ask further questions.

She had just bought a new car and was still getting used to it. We took the journey to Oxford slowly and carefully – far too slowly for me. "Can't you put your foot down?" I kept pleading at periodic intervals.

"Oh, there's no need to hurry," Alison insisted. "We've got plenty of time. We'll be half an hour early as it is, and they're not going to want us to arrive too early and be hanging around, getting in the way!"

I had other thoughts about that. I was sure that they could do with two extra pairs of hands. But I didn't say anything. I just contented myself with staring at the picture of the little dog I was about to meet. I wondered if he would like me. I've always believed that with animals, you can't own them. They have to choose to own you. I remembered the day on which we bought Sam. We went to the kennels and looked into the cage where the Jack Russells were. He saw me, he bounded up to me, and it was obvious that the little puppy wanted to belong to us. But Skipper had been chosen to live with me. He had no say in it, and I hoped we would get on.

"I hope you're going to be able to find this Centre," Alison said.

"Oh, yes." I had spent nights memorising the map, and felt very confident as I directed her off the M40.

"Are you sure it's here? I thought it was in Oxford." I explained that it was on the outskirts of Oxford at Chinnor. As we drove through the lovely countryside, I couldn't think of a better place to train dogs.

For once, my directions were accurate and we soon arrived at the Training Centre. As soon as Alison had parked the car, I literally sprinted to the front door, hardly bothering to take in the pre-fabricated building designed to look like a normal house or bungalow. When I rang the bell, Alison said she could hear a lot of dogs racing towards the door, and then racing towards their respective owners. There were a number of different doorbells, and I only hoped that I had rung the right one. Later, Tony Blunt, the training officer, explained that there were several different doorbells because each dog is trained to respond to the sound of its future owner's bell.

The door opened and Gillian greeted us. We were among the first people to arrive. Alison grinned and gave me an "I told you so" look.

"Would you like a coffee?" Gillian enquired.

"Oh, yes please," said Alison.

I was more interested in meeting Skipper, but I thought it would be impolite to refuse, so we sat down, and I talked to a young man next to me.

He was one of the first recipients of a Hearing Dog and his dog had been sponsored by the viewers of *Pebble Mill at One*. He used sign language, and I asked him if his dog had been of much help to him. "Oh, yes," he replied. "Before the dog came, I was very isolated and cut off. But now I have the dog, my whole life has changed. I don't feel deaf any more."

On the other side of me was an elderly lady with a little chihuahua. "Is that a Hearing Dog?" I asked.

The friend she was with explained that indeed he was, and his name was Scampy. Scampy's owner was deaf and registered blind. When she had had to go into a home, her Guide Dog for the Blind was too big to go with her and had to be taken away. This had made her very withdrawn and the concerned warden of the home eventually wrote to HDFD in the hope that they could provide her with a small Hearing Dog. Scampy had obviously made a great difference to his owner, because she was happily hugging him, her contact with the everyday world resumed.

I asked Tony why most of the dogs they trained were mongrels and he explained that it was because they got most of their dogs from animal rescue centres. "They also have the advantage," Tony went on, "of being less prone to the congenital defects that pedigrees suffer from as a result of overbreeding. They are intelligent, and perhaps inclined to use their initiative more than most dogs."

"Is that very important?" I asked.

"A Hearing Dog will sometimes have to decipher whether a sound is a routine, everyday sound, or something that is important to its deaf owner. The dogs respond to the sounds that they are trained to respond to, but many will use their initiative and respond to other sounds. If you have confidence in Skipper and build up a good relationship with him, you will find that he will help you in many different ways."

Some months after he was eventually placed with me, Skipper gave me a perfect illustration of what Tony meant. He came rushing up one day and led me towards the front-door. But as I opened it, he didn't wag his tail for a friend, or sniff suspiciously for a stranger; instead, he walked straight out of the door and led me to a car parked beside my house. "What is it?" I asked him. He looked adamantly at the car. "Silly dog," I scolded, dragging him back into the house by the collar. I shut the door, but once again Skipper came and got me and led me to the door, and then to the car. Luckily, there was a passer-by, so I asked him if there was a funny noise anywhere.

"Oh yes," he replied. "The alarm on that car is deafening everybody. Can't you hear it?"

"Oh yes," I lied, feeling in touch with things, "I just wondered where the noise was coming from." When the man had gone, I hugged the clever Skipper and richly rewarded him with a lump of cheese.

Now I kept plying Tony with questions. "But how do you decide which ones will make good Hearing Dogs when you see them in a kennel, or somewhere?"

"Well, what I do," Tony explained, "is to take along a collection of things that make noises – a rattle, squeaky toy etc. and see if the dog reacts to them at all."

"A lot of people must wonder what on earth you're doing," Alison joked.

"Yes, I suppose they must," replied Tony, who hadn't thought of that before.

"So when a dog reacts well to these sounds, what else must it do to qualify?" I asked.

"I will take it for a walk and see if it is reasonably placid and good-natured, and if it is, then I'll bring it back to the Centre for a two-week trial period. During that time we'll see how it is with children, and if it has any hang-ups that could affect its ability to perform as a Hearing Dog. For example, the dog might have a fear of cars, or Saturday-morning-shopping streets. If, after these tests, the dog is all right, we keep it, if not, it goes back and gets another home."

Another visitor was Jane, who had just gone deaf. Going deaf in adult life is a traumatic experience. Suddenly, family and friends can no longer communicate with you and you feel very cut off. A person who has gone deaf in later life is frequently unwilling to accept flashing doorbells or vibrating alarm clocks or anything else to remind them that they are in a deaf and alien world. Jane did not want these, but when she was given her Hearing Dog, Benjy, her confidence returned and her communication with the hearing world started again. She was able to take Benjy for walks, she told me, and because she had to explain to other dog-owners what Benjy was, they were patient and realised that lip-reading for her was not a skill acquired from child-hood, but a very strenuous and difficult thing. Walking the dog, they had all the time and patience in the world to talk to her. Friends were able to call round again and use her doorbell. Benjy also gave them a talking point. It saved the embarrassing problem of bringing up her deafness.

Many of the people with Hearing Dogs were elderly. "I felt so scared on my own," one lady confided to me. "I couldn't hear the door, so my daughter gave me a flashing thing, but I couldn't be getting on with it. My dog makes me feel so safe now, living on my own. He keeps me in touch with everything around me."

I had never, until then, realised that a Hearing Dog could be invaluable to elderly people who go deaf in old age and feel very confused and vulnerable when they can't work modern technical aids, even hearing-aids. But they may have always been used to looking after pets. To them a Hearing Dog is not only their com-panion, but their ears and security.

Talking to these other owners of Hearing Dogs, all coming from different backgrounds and circumstances, was very interesting for me. However, interesting as it was, I wanted to meet *my* dog, but I didn't like to be rude and ask. I thought I had better wait until Gillian and Tony felt that the time was right to introduce us. All the same, I kept eyeing Tony and looking hopeful. In the end he grinned and said, "I think you want to meet your dog."

"I'd rather like to," I replied politely, getting up, all ready to charge out to the kennel.

"You sit here," said Tony. "I think it's better if you meet here. I'll go and get him."

When the door opened next, a boisterous Jack Russell puppy raced into the room.

"Skipper!" I shouted.

He responded by taking a flying leap onto my lap and licking me. When he had succeeded in removing all my make-up he poked his nose into my handbag and found a packet of chocolate drops I had brought for him.

I felt as if I had known him for ages and he seemed to feel the same. After he had finished the chocolates, he looked up at me as if to say, what next? He took no notice of anyone else in the room. He just seemed to have eyes for me.

Alison couldn't get over this. "When's he going to make a fuss of me?" she kept asking. But he wasn't interested in Alison. "Just as well," she said. "It would have been awful if he'd made a fuss of me and not you."

I took him for a walk round the Centre, in order to try and get to know him, and realised what a lovely place it was. There was an air of peacefulness about it with the kennels overlooking the orchard. What a lovely place to train the dogs, I kept thinking.

Skipper and I had barely had a chance to get to know each other when we were ushered to pose for press photos with the other dog-owners. We lined up on the green in the orchard with a motley assortment of mongrels, Border Collies and the odd Labrador. We were a very varied bunch – all age groups, from some elderly people to Robert and myself, who were the youngest people there.

Skipper was a real professional about posing. Later, I discovered he has a passion for having his photo taken or being filmed. He sat up straight, pricked his ears and smiled into the cameras. And didn't the photographers love him! "Can you get him to whisper in your ear?" an enthusiastic photographer asked me. Whispering in a deaf owner's ear did not seem to me quite the most intelligent thing for a Hearing Dog to do, but I was so happy that day I didn't think, and I obligingly wedged a chocolate drop into my hearing-aid. To the photographers' delight, Skipper nibbled at the chocolate drop, and I did my best to stop myself from giggling because it was so ticklish.

Eventually, the press session ended, and I went to talk to Robert. Pepper was a Border Collie who Robert hoped would not only be his ears but also replace a much-loved dog who had recently died. Robert had brought his friend Russell with him and, all being of the same age, we got on very well. As Gillian and Tony still seemed tied up with the press people, we decided to take our dogs for a short walk before lunch and Jane and Benjy came too.

I was a bit nervous, because I hadn't asked Gillian and Tony if it was all right. We walked down the road to a field where Robert and Jane let Pepper and Benjy off their leads. I was reluctant to let Skipper off, because I hardly knew him. What if he wouldn't come back to me? I had visions of him running down the road back to the kennels and getting run over. "You must let him off the lead," said Jane. "It's very unkind. I always let Benjy off the lead."

Because Skipper and I were getting along so well, Jane didn't realise that we had only met for the first time half an hour ago. I let him go, praying that he would stay close to Benjy and Pepper and come back to me. But to my relief when I called his name, he came bounding up, and I rewarded him with a chocolate drop. After that, every time I called him, he couldn't come fast enough. In fact, I thought that he was coming back quicker than Benjy or Pepper, so I was really chuffed!

As the time went on, I realised that Skipper and I were a match made in heaven. He never left my side and he wasn't even on the lead. He kept looking up at me with adoring, penetrating black eyes. Friends of mine often say that they can feel Skipper's gaze, and all during that first morning I felt it on me.

At lunch-time he became a little scrounger as the food was passed around and he began to wander through the guests, hopeful of getting an odd scrap. "You mustn't feed him," Tony explained to me. "He's got to learn to associate food with reward, as part of his training." So I made a conscientious effort not to give him anything, and didn't dare mention to Tony that I'd been buying his friendship with chocolate drops earlier.

I don't think that Skipper was very pleased about not being fed, and I did notice, out of the corner of my eye, that someone else was feeding him. Oh well, I thought, it's our first meeting, almost as if it's his birthday. I won't say anything.

"Always give him a chocolate drop after he's answered the phone or the doorbell," I was told at first. But now Skipper doesn't want the chocolate drop. He seems to do his job because he loves doing it, not for reward. Even if people do spoil him at parties and give him sausages and chicken, it's always me he returns to. The bond forged that day was definitely a bond that was to endure throughout our lives together.

After a Hearing Dog has been trained and placed with its owner, it goes through a three-month trial period during which Tony Blunt and Gillian are in constant contact, ironing out any problems and seeing that dog and owner are working well together. After the three months, the dogs which qualify, or perhaps I should say the recipients who qualify as owners of Hearing Dogs, are awarded an orange lead and collar for their dog and a certificate. Unlike Guide Dogs for the Blind, Hearing Dogs don't have a harness, but they can be distinguished by their bright orange lead and collar. The certificate is signed by Tony and stamped by the Centre. This certificate is invaluable to carry round with you, since Hearing Dogs can come in all shapes and sizes, so people like BR guards or shop owners have difficulty in recognising them as guide dogs and try to bar their entry. It is to be hoped that, as they become more widely recognised and known, the orange lead and collar, together with the certificate, will dispel any doubts people may have about a Hearing Dog's credentials.

As I watched the presentation of the orange leads and collars to some other doggy graduates, I longed for the day when Skipper would get his. He still looked very puppyish, with long legs for a Jack Russell and his undocked tail weighing him down. His paws were large and puppyish too. He seemed so much of a baby, I wondered if he'd ever qualify for his orange lead and collar as he sat beside me and eyed the ceremony.

Now I was dreading the end of the open day and having to say goodbye for two whole months. I was one of the last to leave. I gave Skipper a final pat and hug and handed him over to Tony. He trotted out of the door, looking behind him as if to say, I'm going to miss you too.

Alison had had to leave earlier, so I was getting a lift back to London with Robert and Russell who, realising I was upset, got hundreds of photographs out of the dashboard and spent the whole journey showing them to me and chattering, to take my mind off Skipper. This was just as well, otherwise I think that I would have been crying in the back seat.

# 4

# Skipper's Got A Secret

As it turned out, I did not have to wait two months before seeing Skipper again. I was on duty subtitling one Saturday, when there was an urgent phone call for me. Gillian had been invited to appear on the BBC quiz show *I've Got a Secret*. On this show a celebrity panel has to guess the unusual, interesting or amazing secrets of the various guests. As Gillian's secret was, of course, "I train Hearing Dogs for the deaf," the producer decided he wanted a dog who was undergoing training to appear on the show after the panel had done their guessing. Skipper had been picked. Now someone was needed at short notice to walk Skipper on and, as I was his future owner and on the BBC premises, I was asked if I would do it.

What I didn't realise was that I had to do it there and then! "Could you come straight away," the programme researcher pleaded. "We're only in the Bush Theatre down the road from you."

My hair needed washing, and as it was a Saturday I was wearing old clothes. There was no way that I would appear on television in plimsolls and without make-up. I was sure they didn't want someone in jeans to walk the dog on.

"Well, I can't come for an hour," I lied. "Someone has to come and replace me because I'm on duty, and I'll have to ring them up and they'll have to come in, so do you mind giving me an hour and a half?"

The programme researcher just seemed relieved I'd agreed to do it. "All right, come to the Television Theatre in Shepherd's Bush Green when you can. But please make that as quick as possible."

Luckily, I was not the only subtitler on duty that day. I bribed Ruth with offers to do all her late shifts that week if she would stay on and work that evening. When I explained to her what had happened, that Skipper was actually in London appearing on a television programme, she was only too pleased to help out. She wished me luck and said to try and bring Skipper back to meet her afterwards.

I hailed a taxi, despite the fact that I only live ten minutes' walk from Television Centre, dived into the bathroom, washed my hair, slapped on some make-up, changed into my best dress and then got another taxi back to the television studio, all of fifteen minutes' walk away.

I wondered if Skipper would recognise me. I couldn't wait to see him. What a shame there'd been no time to buy him a present.

The security man at the Television Theatre escorted me to a dressing-room. I'd never seen behind the scenes at Television Centre, Wood Lane, despite having worked there for two years, and to go into a dressing-room at the Bush Theatre was an experience I'll never forget – especially the moment when I opened the door and Skipper came up, wagging his tail, delighted to see me.

Sitting in a chair was Gillian, being made up for her big moment. "I'm *so* glad you could come," she said. "I was terribly worried about Skipper. I thought if someone walked him on who didn't know him, he might misbehave. I just hope he's not going to disgrace himself," she added.

"Never mind," I said. "If there's time, I'll take him for a walk first."

"That's just the problem," Gillian wailed. "We *can't* take Skipper for a walk in case one of the panel sees him and guesses my secret too quickly when they are given the initial clue. He's got to keep a very low profile, and we've been here since eleven o'clock this morning."

I felt sorry for Skipper, but he didn't seem at all bothered. He was pleased to see me and even more pleased when his dinner was brought in. When I'd got over my delight at seeing him again, I had time to begin to feel nervous on my own account, but the programme researcher, was very reassuring and took Skipper and me along to be briefed by the programme's presenter, Tom O'Connor. "I'm so pleased that you could help us out," he said. "We really do appreciate it, and it was very kind of you to come at such short notice."

I assured him that it was no trouble at all and that I was only too delighted to see Skipper again, even if it meant appearing on television!

"Oh, that's nothing to worry about," Tom reassured me. "All you have to do is walk Skipper on."

"But how will I know when to do it?" I asked.

"Don't worry," the stage manager said. "I'll get somebody to stand behind you and give you a push. Then you walk up these steps, and go over to Gillian."

I practised that first, just to make sure that I'd got it right.

"And then," said Tom, "I will ask you a few questions about Skipper, and in case you're nervous at the time and can't lip-read me, we'll discuss the questions now. I think I should ask you what he's going to do for you and how he's going to help you."

I explained about the alarm clocks and doorbells and telephones, and mentioned how he would also be trained to alert me to fire-alarms and burglars.

"I think that's a very important point," said Tom. "We'll definitely bring that up." He also said that he thought he should ask me what my job was. People would then know that Skipper was actually going to come to the BBC and work in an office and give me independence at work.

"Will the panel ask me any questions?" I inquired.

"Would you like them to?"

"Not really," I replied, thinking that I would be very, very nervous.

"That's all right, then," said Tom. "I'll make sure that I ask all the questions, and we'll only discuss the questions we've already talked about now."

I felt much more confident as I returned to Gillian who was still fretting about Skipper disgracing himself on the studio floor.

"Don't worry," said the stage manager philosophically. "If he does cock his leg while he's on the set, this programme will just be the Christmas show."

That cheered me up, but I don't think it helped Gillian. "It's Hearing Dogs' reputation," she kept saying, "and nobody's going to realise that he's been cooped up in this building since eleven o'clock."

I had more confidence in Skipper, and he proved that my faith in him was justified. He might have been born to work in a television studio. He didn't bark while the show was being recorded, and he became one of the few dogs not to foul a studio – so much for being in the Christmas show!

When the audience heard what Gillian's secret was, she was greeted with very warm applause. This set the panel on the right track. Their clue was "Sounds like my pet subject," and they immediately ruled out animal experiments because of the audience's warm reaction. They started asking questions about training animals and working in a circus. Jan Leeming was on the panel, and Skipper had appeared on *News Review* a few weeks earlier in some film of the Training Centre, so I was worried that she would catch on too soon. Anneka Rice eventually suggested Guide Dogs for the Blind and when this was turned down, Jan suggested HDFD, which was correct.

When it was time for us to go on, Skipper must have heard his name called, because before I felt a kindly push from behind, he was pulling me forward. He doesn't understand what stage fright is, I thought, as I followed. He made a bee-line for Gillian, and she decided that she would pick him up to avoid any accidents on the studio floor.

"What kind of a dog is he?" Tom O'Connor asked me.

"I think he's pretending to be a Jack Russell," I replied. "He's really too long and tall, and most Jack Russells have a short tail."

Tom continued to ask me the questions we had prepared beforehand. Skipper was blissfully upstaging both of us by licking Jan Leeming's make-up off. "Let's hope he doesn't lick the burglars!" Tom quipped to the studio audience.

Later, Skipper was to prove that Tom's fears were ill-founded and that he would be well able to distinguish burglars from friendly lady newsreaders. One day at home, Skipper came up to me, tapped me on the leg, and ran towards the kitchen window, growling and snarling. I followed him, wondering what on earth it could be. He kept running towards the back window of my flat, still growling and snarling, and I decided that I had better go down and investigate. I walked very cautiously round to the back of the house to discover that my downstairs neighbour had forgotten his key and was trying to break through his own window. Skipper was obviously never going to let me down with burglars.

After *I've Got a Secret* had been recorded, I took Skipper onto Shepherd's Bush Green, where he thankfully cocked his leg! He didn't seem very happy in the city. I think he was a bit scared by all the traffic. Shepherd's Bush is a far cry from the quiet countryside of Chinnor and Stow-on-the-Wold. I hoped he was going to adapt to city life.

When I got back to the studio, I confided my fears to Gillian. "Don't worry," she said. "What I'm going to suggest is that Skipper stays the weekend with you, and you can get to know each other – not that you two need to. And then, if it's all right, I could come and collect him on Monday morning."

"Oh, I can bring him back to Chinnor on Monday morning," I replied, delighted.

"Would you really?" said Gillian. "That would save

me a lot of trouble, and you could have another look at the Training Centre. But," she warned me, "don't worry if he doesn't answer telephones and door bells this weekend. After all, he has got two more months' training to go. Don't expect too much of him, but if he does respond to anything, reward him."

Gillian had brought his food and his bowl with her. All I had to do was take care of him. I was so excited. Skipper was coming to stay with me for the weekend. I wanted to take him over straight away and introduce him to Ruth, but first of all, there was the after-show party for all guests and panel of *I've Got a Secret*. Everybody made a fuss of Skipper and Tom O'Connor came and asked a lot more questions about Hearing Dogs. Since then he has held coffee mornings and raised a considerable amount of money for Hearing Dogs. A few years later, a journalist colleague of mine, writing for a magazine for the deaf, was doing some celebrity interviews, and when she talked to Tom O'Connor, he mentioned meeting Skipper and me on *I've Got a Secret*, and said that meeting us had been the start of his concern for deaf people. That meant a lot to me, to think that Skipper had influenced somebody like Tom.

The other guests on the show were as interested as the panel. One of the guests was Richard Stilgoe, whose secret was, "I lived in a hearse." Apparently, when he was a penniless actor he really did live in a hearse! He asked a lot of questions about Skipper, about how I learned to lip-read, and what it meant to be deaf, and we talked for a long time. Like Tom O'Connor, he was not to forget that evening. A year later a letter arrived from Hodder and Stoughton saying that Richard Stilgoe had written to them suggesting I write a book about my experiences as a deaf person, and with Skipper. It was because of this meeting that evening that the whole idea of writing this book was conceived.

The other guests on the show were a really interesting mixture of people. There was the painter, Heath Robinson's daughter, and a man who had posed in a girlie calendar in a suspender belt! Mr Universe from

1950, the man who held the world record for keeping a
ferret in his pocket, a lady who had danced with Fred
Astaire and a man who had been locked in Broadmoor
for an hour by mistake. It was fascinating to talk to all
these people, and they were very patient and understanding of my problem.

Skipper was fed up. He was tired; he'd had a long
day. While I was chatting, he just flopped down on the
floor. But Skipper's day was far from over. Gillian and
I were sent off in a taxi, she to her car and me to
Television Centre. We decided to drop Gillian off first,
and when she got out of the taxi Skipper stood up on his
hind legs and peered anxiously out of the rear window as
we drove away, as if to say, where's she gone? Why am
I left with you? But when we got to Television Centre,
he got out of the taxi with an air of expectation. It was
almost as if he knew that he was going to work there.
As he walked down the corridors to the Subtitling Unit,
he was taking in his surroundings, and he looked up
as if to say, I think I know I'm going to like working
here.

We opened the door, and there was Ruth, about to
go home. "I thought you were never coming," she said,
as she donned an old brown raincoat. The raincoat was
bulky and probably crackled alarmingly. Skipper took
one look and nearly fled out of the office. There must
have been something about raincoats in his puppy past.
But as soon as Ruth took the raincoat off, Skipper went
to say hello, and a very firm friendship was forged
between them that evening. Skipper has always had a
special affection for Ruth. It's as if he knows that Ruth
has been one of the people who has helped me most. If
it wasn't for Ruth I wouldn't have started subtitling.
Ruth helped to establish my career and Skipper knows
that.

It has always amazed me how resilient Skipper is,
how easily he takes new situations in his stride and
adapts to new places. Within minutes of meeting Ruth,
he was quite at home in Television Centre, and when
he left the building and went home to my small flat, after

some initial sniffing around and getting his bearings, he was equally at home there. He sat down on the sofa, and curled up, as if to say, this is where I'm going to sleep. I gave him a blanket, which he gratefully made into a bed. One of Skipper's most endearing habits is the way he makes his own bed. You give him a blanket and he forms it into a semi-circle and proceeds to curl up in the middle. Sometimes he is dissatisfied with the way he's made his bed and has to make it again. I spent a happy five minutes, watching him making his bed and settling down for the night.

I could hardly get to sleep that night. I kept staring at him on the sofa. I couldn't believe that he was there. It was so comforting to have another presence in the flat. Normally, I am very scared of the dark and I always sleep with the light on. Maybe it's because I know that in the dark I have no means of communication. But that night I felt extra confident and turned off the light. I also set the alarm clock, to see if Skipper would answer it.

The next morning, I was woken up by Skipper jumping onto my bed and licking my face. Gosh! I thought, he's answered the alarm clock! So I duly rewarded him with a chocolate drop. Only after he had eaten it and was happily smacking his lips, did I look at the clock. It was seven and I had set the alarm for nine! It occurred to me that perhaps he was used to being fed at that time, but I sent him to bed again and went back to sleep. The next time he woke me up it really was nine o'clock, so I rewarded him by giving him *two* chocolate drops and hoped that he'd get the message that waking-up time was when the alarm went off, and not when his tummy decided it was breakfast-time.

That Sunday with Skipper was one of the happiest days of my life. I spent the whole day walking him in the park and by the end of it he seemed to be less bothered by London and its traffic. He made friends with Tessa and Flash, two dogs in the park, and played with them, running round and round in circles. Their owners came up to talk to me and I was able to tell them about Skipper being a Hearing Dog. They were very

45

interested, keen to talk to me, and understanding when I misheard them sometimes. It occurred to me that I was going to meet a lot of people through Skipper. Not only had I acquired a canine friend, but through him I would find other friends.

The day passed all too quickly, and once again Skipper made his bed on the sofa. I set the alarm clock for eight, knowing that the next day I would be taking him back. I wondered if he'd answer the alarm or his tummy. I need not have worried. When the alarm went off, there was Skipper jumping on me and licking my face. He'd obviously learnt his lesson of the day before.

Sadly I drove Skipper back to Chinnor to complete his education. For about fifteen minutes, I watched him charge round the Centre, chasing a rubber bone and playing with the other trainee dogs. It was lovely to see how happy and relaxed they were. Underneath the responsible Hearing Dog was a happy, playful little mongrel and now I was counting the days until he'd be mine for good.

# 5

## Skipper At The Centre

Gillian was to bring Skipper on a Friday and leave him to settle with me over the weekend. Then on the Monday she would come back and start teaching him to associate the sounds that he had learnt at the Centre with me.

"I'll ring you at work," she wrote, "then you won't have to take a whole day off and you'll know that I have arrived." I didn't get much work done that morning! A little before lunch-time, Gillian rang to say that she was waiting outside my flat.

"I'll sort out the machine; you just go," said Ruth when she heard. I took up her offer, and couldn't drive home fast enough.

Outside my flat there was Gillian with Skipper, who was sitting patiently by the door. When I arrived he raced to meet me as if to say, why weren't you here to welcome me? Don't you know how to welcome someone? Never mind, I'll show you. To this day Skipper's wagging tail and high-flying welcome leaps are something our friends wish that they could politely avoid.

I unlocked the front-door and Skipper hurtled up the stairs to the door of my flat which he recognised from his previous visit. "You can't wait to show me your new home, can you?" said Gillian following him up the stairs. "He's been waiting to come all morning. We bathed him and he immediately went and stood by my car as if he knew." Gillian looked round the flat and laughed. "I've brought you a bowl and lead etc., but it looks like you don't need anything. Lucky little dog." Skipper was already sitting on his blanket on the sofa looking at

47

Gillian as if to say, make yourself at home in my house. "I was going to spend the afternoon making sure he settled down all right, but it doesn't look as if you two need me any more today. So I'll see you Monday."

Almost as soon as Gillian had gone I was aware of a presence. Two bright brown eyes were glued on me. Twenty-four hours a day I feel Skipper's presence. In the morning when he wakes me up, it is there. He watches me put on my make-up before I go to work and I can feel his eyes saying too much eye-shadow, or very nice. All day at work I feel his supportive presence, and even in the evening when he curls up tired after a day's work, he keeps one sleepy eye open. He is always alert, and as soon as a sound goes off he springs into action, racing to tap my leg and then racing off to the source of the noise. Occasionally on a bad day at work he might have a leisurely stretch before alerting me, but he is always there and he gives me great confidence.

Confidence is the secret to a good working relationship with a guide dog, be it a Hearing Dog or a Guide Dog for the Blind. I have confidence in Skipper and always rely on him, and he knows it and works well for me, feeling important. I remember meeting a blind couple in Wales, when I was researching a *Songs of Praise*. They each had a Guide Dog and both dogs worked extremely well for them. They were fascinated to hear about Skipper and we were soon swopping stories about our dogs. "Blind people are not always completely blind," they told me. "Some of us see things in shades of light and dark, or may not see anything but a very, very bright light. Just as you have a little residual hearing, we have some residual sight."

The parallels between degrees of sight and hearing are amazing. Few people are completely deaf. My high-powered Phonac hearing-aids make an under-water garble, with the odd words becoming distinctive. The better I know somebody, the more words become clear, especially if they have a high-pitched voice. I can get a fair amount of what my mother says. What I don't understand I supplement with lip-reading. I wear my aids most of the time now, as a garbled, incoherent sound is better than nothing. When I first got them I couldn't make out words and I just wore them because a faint garble was better than a silent world with an occasional whisper. But I found that with practice and by getting to know people I recognised occasional words. However limited they are, my aids are a comfort and a contact. So I wear them when there are people around, but not when I'm alone, because they make me feel tired. In the company of friends I know well, I don't wear them and I lip-read.

I wear the aids in both ears. I hear most in my left ear – it takes an unusually loud sound, and the aid, for my right ear to hear anything. Even a loud fire-alarm would be part of the porridge of sound, and a fire-alarm without my hearing-aids on would be silence, or if I was concentrating, an indistinguishable far-away whisper.

I cannot distinguish sounds – they are part of the garble; so even with the hearing-aids, Skipper is essential and invaluable, and I would never dream of letting him know that I can sometimes hear my mother. It would confuse him horribly. The blind couple were aware of the same problem. "Sometimes we can see a car with very bright headlights, but we never let the dogs know that." We certainly need our dogs. Seeing the occasional bright light or hearing the odd word or sound by using intense concentration is not something that you can do all day all the time, and you do still miss out on ninety-nine per cent of the other sounds and sights that the dogs alert you to.

Skipper had trust in me, and settled down very quickly. It was only a few hours since Gillian had left when he raced up and tapped my knee. "What is it?" I asked, doing what Gillian had told me to do. He trotted towards my phone and stood beside it. "Good boy," I said, rewarding him with a Good-Boy Choc drop as Gillian had also told me to do.

Then I answered the phone. "It's Mummy," said a high-pitched voice that I was so well tuned into. "I thought I'd give Skipper some practice! Come and see us. We want to meet him." I replied that we'd go down to the South Coast and see them the next day.

Saturday morning I was suddenly woken by what felt like a heavy weight falling on my stomach. Winded, I opened my eyes to a wet doggy tongue on my face. What a way to be woken up! "Thank you," I said, "but no more flying leaps, please!" Thankfully, Skipper has gradually become more gentle at this delicate hour of the day.

After a long walk in the park, he jumped in my car and sat on his blanket on the back seat. As I drove out of London, I could see him out of the corner of the car rear mirror happily looking out of the window, until he eventually settled down. As soon as we arrived, mum and dad rushed out to the car. "We can't wait to meet him!" they shouted. A good reception committee is something that Skipper always appreciates and their enthusiastic welcome put them straight into his good books. If that didn't, the smell of home-made baking in the kitchen did! He rushed straight into the kitchen, his chops drooling. "I've cooked him some chicken for his supper as a coming-home present. Can he have it?" mum confided. I told Skipper to look forward to a gourmet supper. He gave me his "can't I have it now" look, then followed dad into the garden for a game. He was obviously a hit.

To help pass the time until his gourmet dinner, we took him for a walk on the Downs. Skipper couldn't get over the vast open space and raced round and round us; he seemed tireless. Every time he saw another dog, he charged up to it in leaps and bounds. Not many dogs were amused by this boisterous greeting and declined to play with him. "Poor thing," said dad throwing a stick for him. By chance, the stick fell next to a large cow pat that Skipper took one look at and happily rolled in. This seemed to give him the confidence to approach other dogs again and, if they had avoided him the first time, they definitely gave him the cold shoulder now! But at least the walk seemed to tire him out and it certainly gave him an appetite for his chicken, which he gulped down after his second bath in two days.

Mum, dad and I were having our own dinner when Skipper came and gently nudged my knee. "What is it?" I asked. He trotted into the hall and stopped at the middle of the wall. Mum and dad followed us to see Skipper in action. "What is it?" I asked again, convinced that the wall couldn't make a noise, feeling embarrassed because mum and dad were entitled to a better exhibition than this. But Skipper refused to budge.

Suddenly dad ran into the kitchen and answered the phone. I was about to tell Skipper off, but mum came to his rescue. "The phone sounds out in the hall as there's a bell out here too, and this has obviously confused him." I gave Skipper his reward by the phone and after a while he learnt to associate the sound with where the reward (and the phone) was. "What a clever boy you are!" said mum, hugging the smug-looking Skipper. "You must send me the addresses of the ladies who sponsored him."

I explained that one lady wished to remain anonymous, but gave her Stella Binns' address, which I knew by heart as I had written a long letter of introduction and thanks the day after I had first met Skipper at Chinnor.

Mum and dad's house was soon to become Skipper's second home. "You can come here any time," dad told him, as he waved us out of the drive that evening. "And if your mistress goes away you must come here for a holiday." Skipper grinned his happy doggy grin as if to say, and we'll go for walks and find lots of cow pats, then went to sleep on the back seat, an exhausted dog.

Monday morning soon arrived and I was treated to another rude awakening. After breakfast, a gentle paw nudged me and Skipper led me to the door. Why can't he be gentle like this when he wakes me up? I mused. It was Gillian. "You clever dog!" she said as she greeted Skipper. She had taken my spare keys with her in case she needed them to get in, but was pleased not to have to use them.

I told her how well he had done and that he was already responding to sounds. "Does this always happen?" I asked.

"No, it's very rare for a dog instantly to associate with its new owner what it has learnt at the Centre with its trainer, and that's what I usually help you both to do this week, but I see I'm going to be redundant! And the fact that you have confidence in him helps. A dog knows when someone hasn't got confidence in it and starts to play up." However, Gillian checked Skipper's response to various sounds before she accepted that his cleverness and my confidence in him had made her week with us plain sailing.

"What we'll do," she explained, "is to go and visit your vet, so that he can check Skipper up, and you and Skipper can get to know him. Also, as Skipper has to work in the office, I'd better settle him in there as he may have trouble with all the various phones." We went to see the family vet who had nursed my dog Sam through many an illness in his long old age. He was very interested to meet Skipper, as he had already heard about Hearing Dogs from a veterinary colleague who was on the committee. Gillian explained to us both that Hearing Dogs, like Guide Dogs for the Blind, received two check-ups a year and free injections annually. Our vet examined Skipper, pronounced him fighting fit and added that he only expected to see him twice a year.

It was now time to take Skipper to work at Television Centre. I parked my car in the carpark and proudly walked Skipper towards the building. "You can't take that dog in!" said the commissionaire on the gate.

"But he's my Hearing Dog!" I exclaimed. "Haven't Personnel told you about him? It's all official."

The commissionaire said he'd have to ring Personnel. We waited. Then all was well. "You weren't expected until later in the week and the memo is still on its way." Skipper looked up as if to say, none of you lot thought that I would be so clever, did you? Soon all the commissionaires were making a fuss of him. Every morning Skipper gives them a special morning grin and every evening, he gives them a goodnight grin and never has to show his staff status!

Gillian couldn't get over Television Centre. "Look, Skipper, there's Terry Wogan," she whispered.

I assured Gillian that the novelty of the Centre was something you soon took for granted. I then remembered my first day there two years previously. I had applied for a job as a subtitler in Ceefax and been amazed when I actually got a BBC interview. As a child, television was mostly meaningless to me before I developed my communication skills. But every night the family used to sit around the screen and watch it – it was like a deity. As I wasn't allowed to talk during this serious televiewing, I watched too, making up my own stories to supplement the pictures. Then gran would walk me down to the Centre, which was not far from our flat, and explain that the pictures on the TV came from there. It was magic: the Centre was a fairy castle to me, where magicians lived, and I wanted to be one.

The board for the Ceefax job went well but they thought I was too deaf to subtitle, so at first offered me a clerical job in the department. That wasn't what I wanted, and as I couldn't type or do shorthand, I was not really geared to it. Nevertheless, it was a BBC job, so I accepted, and will always remember the first day, walking into Television Centre from Wood Lane, the palace of my dreams.

If the atmosphere had at first overawed Gillian and me, it did not have much effect on Skipper, who happily trotted behind us as if there was nothing unusual about the place. Some people gave him a few looks, but said nothing. Everybody in Subtitling was really pleased to see him. "We weren't expecting him until later on in the week," Sue, the Chief Subtitler exclaimed.

I explained about Skipper being so precocious.

"Clever doggie. Congratulations, and welcome to subtitling!" said Sue patting him enthusiastically.

"Is there anything that we must do to help him?" Ruth asked Gillian.

"Yes," Gillian replied. "You must never feed him or

play with him in the office, because he must learn to respond to Kerena only. When he answers the phone for her, she will reward him, so it's better to ignore him. It would also help if you could wait and let Skipper tell Kerena her phone's ringing, or he might get confused and not tell her when she is on her own."

Gillian's advice certainly helped establish a working relationship with Skipper. Skipper has always had his own phone with a different ring from the others, so that everyone else can answer their phones without waiting for him to give the go-ahead. As for not making a fuss of him, we stuck to Gillian's advice for the first six months, but there's now such a strong bond between him and me that, although he's spoilt rotten by everyone else, it doesn't confuse him one bit or stop him doing his job for me.

Meanwhile, that first day in the office turned out to be a busy one. "I'm glad you're here," Sue commented. "Your *Hi-de-Hi* has arrived and we are getting pushed, so it would be nice to have that out of the way."

"Do you mind subtitling with me?" I asked Gillian, "Or would you rather I worked with you and Skipper?"

"It's better that you do whatever you usually do and I'll watch," she said. "Besides, I'd love to see how subtitling is done, and meanwhile, every so often I'll make a sound for Skipper to respond to."

We placed Skipper's basket beside my machine and I began to tell Gillian a little about subtitling. "It takes about thirty hours to subtitle an hour's programme," I explained. "We can't just type in what's said because nobody can read as fast as people talk, and as some viewers are elderly and read slowly, and some have impaired reading-ability because of their deafness, we take out about a third of what's being said, depending on how slowly the person speaks."

"And you use different colour text to distinguish between characters, don't you?" Gillian said. "I've seen your subtitles when I've been placing dogs."

"That's right. Usually we use black backgrounds, but

coloured ones are given to monsters and non-human characters. It makes it more fun for kids."

"But how do you subtitle if you can't hear?" Gillian asked. "How did you learn?"

I explained that I soon got bored with the clerical job I was doing and was convinced that I could subtitle. There is a script and a cassette of the programme, and it seemed to me that all I had to do was to put words and pictures together.

Ruth and Irene were most supportive. "Ask Sue if you can have a go at subtitling in your spare time and we'll help you," they suggested. Sue agreed, so every evening after work I would have a go, patiently playing the cassette and putting in the words. Whenever the speaker was in the picture I was all right, but when the speech was off screen, I began to run into trouble.

"If only I could tell what was going on off screen," I complained one day. Peter, one of our engineers, overheard and answered my prayers. He went to PC Werth, an audiological advisory company and hearing-aid suppliers, and learnt about how my hearing-aids could be linked directly to the sound in the cassette through a special amplifier. But since the sound could go straight from the machine into that amplifier and then into my hearing-aid, no one else would hear the loud volume. He then made me an appropriate device. This was a real breakthrough and I practised for a few weeks.

At first all I heard was noise, but gradually, with the help of the script, and as I got used to the characters in the programmes, I began to get much of what was said off screen. At times I almost gave up, but Ruth and Irene encouraged me, while Sue and David, the Teletext Manager, were delighted and offered to pay me if I did extra subtitling in the evening.

Being deaf myself helped me to be sensitive to what was needed. It is very easy to appear patronising to a deaf person in a subtitle. KNOCK KNOCK put up when it is obvious that there is someone knocking can make a deaf viewer feel at least irritated, at worst humiliated.

This I was very aware of. I was also aware that subtitles can look boring and I had learnt from Angie, my school friend, that nobody speaks in a monotone, so I began to put feeling into my subtitles. "I love you . . . I'll NEVER leave you again," looks more interesting than "I love you. I'll never leave you again." Ruth and Irene told me if I put the emphasis on the wrong word and always checked my programmes to see if I had misheard anything, just as I advised them from a deaf viewer's standpoint. Eventually, either because I was good at subtitling, or so bad at the clerical job – I'm not sure which – I got a full-time subtitling job.

It was useful having Gillian sitting behind me that Monday, as the episode of *Hi-de-Hi* was difficult. Spike, the camp comedian, had decided to become a ventriloquist in this episode, but was not very good at it, and I couldn't tell that.

"Is he a good ventriloquist?" I had to ask Gillian.

"You probably can't hear it," she replied, "but the sound is definitely coming out of his mouth."

"Thanks," I replied. "I'll have a go at showing that in the subtitle somehow." I decided to place the subtitle by Spike's mouth, so nobody could possibly doubt where the sound was coming from.

Subtitling was useful in helping me pick up nuances. Deaf people are often slow to get jokes that are a play on words or colloquialisms. Battle Abbey school had helped me considerably to acquire language, but subtitling really helped me build on it. At first I couldn't understand jokes like "I'm made of wood, but I WOODN'T let that bother you, OAKAY?" Ruth patiently explained these appalling jokes to me and eventually I began to pick them up myself, but always let Ruth or someone check my programme to see if I had missed any.

Gillian enjoyed watching me subtitle, but every now and again she would get up, leave the room, and knock at the door and Skipper would come and tap my knee with his paw and lead me to the door. When the phone rang he would come and get me and take me to whichever phone rang. It was luxury! Previously I had had to subtitle, constantly glancing at the flashing light on the phone, and often losing track of what I was doing, but now I could rely on Skipper, and I was getting more subtitles done because of this.

"You really are working well together. It's wonderful," Gillian commented. "I have to give every dog that I place a progress report, and Skipper is going to get a very good one."

It was just as well that Skipper and I were working well together because his arrival at Television Centre was attracting a great deal of attention. Skipper was one of the first Hearing Dogs to be trained, and he was the first dog to work in an office. He'd only been at work a day when the staff magazine, *Ariel*, arrived to do a feature on him.

"This will explain what he is and why he is here to the other staff," someone from Personnel explained. Skipper loved the attention. He posed for photos like a real professional. The flash-bulb on the camera intrigued him and he couldn't take his bright eyes off it.

A few days after the article appeared a researcher from *SuperStore* came down to the Subtitling Unit. Would Skipper appear on *SuperStore*?

"*SuperStore* is live. What do you think?" I asked Gillian, who was still with us.

"Well, it's up to you, but you must have confidence in Skipper. There will be a lot to distract him in the studio," she warned.

I had a quick think. It would be good publicity for Hearing Dogs and it would appeal to children who might learn how to deal with deaf children in their class. "I'll do it," I said, "but can Gillian come too?"

"Of course," said *SuperStore*. "John Craven will be interviewing you. He'll come and meet you a few days before so that you can prepare the questions in advance."

That was a relief, and Gillian and I agreed that Skipper would call me to answer a phone, a knock at the door and respond to the alarm clock in the studio.

The Friday before the programme was to be broadcast,

Skipper and I went to the studio to meet John Craven. It had been raining and Skipper soon got the watercolour paint that was used to paint the set all over himself, the seats in the studio, John's clothes and mine. "It'll wash off," John assured me.

We agreed we'd start with the phone. "And you had better bring your special amplified phone and one of your printing phones along, because the children will wonder how you use a phone. After we've discussed that we'll do the alarm clock and chat about how Skipper will help you in the home and at work. Then we'll have a knock at the door – Gillian can do that. Then when and if Skipper answers the door she can come in and talk about Hearing Dogs. It'll be a nice piece and we won't let it get too complicated, because it's a children's programme."

Everyone was worried that the noise in the studio would put Skipper off. John had the answer. "Let's have a run through now and get everyone to make as much distracting noise as they can." We did just that and Skipper responded only to what he should to everybody's relief.

Skipper's performance was not the only thing that we had to worry about. Subtitling was only done on recorded programmes, but a new machine that could instantly produce live subtitles was in its development stage under Ruth and Elizabeth's guidance. "I'll subtitle the interview," Ruth volunteered. "It will give Elizabeth and me some good practice for when we do *Blue Peter* live and our own viewers might like to see you and Skipper and understand what's said."

Despite Skipper's promising performance on the Friday, I was still nervous on Saturday. "Don't worry, you'll both be fine," said everybody, feeling relieved that the paint had washed off Skipper, as a multi-coloured dog was not a welcome prospect. As soon as we were on the air, Skipper answered the phone. Then he went and settled down in his basket until the next sound came up. "He's the only member of staff at the BBC to be paid in chocolate drops," John told the young viewers as I rewarded Skipper with a Good-Boy Choc drop. This obviously sparked off the children's imagination, for Skipper received a lot of chocolate drops in the post for weeks afterwards! Many young viewers also sent in donations for Hearing Dogs, and I was delighted that Skipper was such a good ambassador for the scheme. However, some deaf people were less enthusiastic, and among the many warm letters from deaf people, I got a few letters of criticism. "How could you accept a dog that takes £2,500 to train," one deaf person wrote, "when you could have flashing lights and vibrating alarm clocks, and live with a friend instead of living on your own?" I felt rather sad at the lack of understanding and wrote back trying to explain that this often quoted £2,500 is not just the cost of training one dog, but has built into it a contribution towards the running and staffing of the Training Centre. In fact, as the Centre grows, the sponsors get better and better value for their money.

After the *SuperStore* interview, Gillian, Skipper and I were invited to the *SuperStore* reception. There we met Mike and Stella Binns from Loughborough. Stella was one of the people who had raised the money for Skipper and meeting her at last made my day. Stella's day was made when John Craven came over to have a chat and give Skipper a congratulatory pat for doing so well.

The Monday after *SuperStore* Skipper had a phone call from the Identity Unit asking him to go to see them at eleven o'clock. I wondered what on earth they could want him for. Nevertheless I walked him round. As we entered the Unit, I noticed a news film crew, equipped with cameras and lights. "The BBC have decided to give Skipper a BBC identity card to prevent any misunderstanding over his presence here," the lady in the Identity Unit explained. "He's also going to have his own staff number – D00001. Do you think he could sit in the chair and have his photo taken?" I plonked Skipper on the chair and told him to sit. He looked at me as if to say, what's happening? then stared at the camera after the initial flash. The news film crew enthusiastically filmed the proceedings. "*News* want to do a spot on you tomorrow, so we're filming this, and if it's all right we'll film you and Skipper in the office."

I couldn't get over Skipper's amazing newsworthiness and phoned mum to tell her.

"Luckily, I've got the day off work, so I'll video it," she said.

Skipper appeared on the lunch-time *News* the next day and the item was repeated on *John Craven's Newsround*, the *Six O'clock News* and the *Nine O'clock News!* Skipper was famous. Mum had a field day.

But it didn't stop there. I was becoming companion to a celebrity. The next day Gillian contacted me. "Skipper's going to get an award. Heineken Lager saw him on the news and every year they give a special award to something that refreshes something that other things can't get to." This was a very confusing message and Gillian wasn't even sure what Skipper had won. "Never mind what he's won; they're coming to present it to him in the Subtitling Unit next week. Oh, and Hearing Dogs have got one as well, whatever it is!" Everyone was very amused and had visions of Heineken posters of Skipper refreshing the parts that other beers couldn't reach. We hadn't got a clue what he had won and had to wait for the award ceremony to find out.

Heineken arrived in great style. Two hefty men carried two enormous crates of Heineken into the Subtitling Unit. "Is that for Skipper?" asked Sharon, imagining a rather drunk, pot-bellied Jack Russell.

"One crate for him; one crate for Hearing Dogs," the man replied.

"I'll drink Skipper's beer," I assured Sharon, "and when we've run out of inspiration subtitling, we'll all drink it!"

The beer was not the only thing that arrived. Two attractive blonde models dressed in immaculate white Heineken sweat-shirts and ski pants arrived and proceeded to squirt hair-spray and perfume all over themselves. "This is all for your benefit," I whispered to Skipper, trying very hard to keep a straight face. Sharon and Ruth had already disappeared, unable to control their giggles. Gillian had come down for the ceremony and was also highly amused.

Finally, two male executives arrived carrying two inscribed brass cubes. Gillian was awarded one with the inscription "To Hearing Dogs for refreshing work with the deaf". And Skipper's read "For refreshing the lives of the deaf". Despite my amusement, I was very touched and proud. It was wonderful that Heineken had seen and appreciated the work done by Hearing Dogs and the Subtitling Unit and found this way to honour it.

The interest that Skipper's arrival at the BBC had generated was good publicity for Hearing Dogs and great fun. I did feel privileged to own one of the first Hearing Dogs for the Deaf. But being a pioneer can have its drawbacks. After all, people still have to be educated about Hearing Dogs.

I'd drunk so much of Skipper's Heineken that I decided not to drive home and got the bus instead. On the bus I noticed a sign saying "Guide Dogs travel free". So, when the conductor came for Skipper's fare, I explained about him being a Hearing Dog and asked if he could travel free. The conductor remembered seeing him on the *News* and was very sympathetic, but when he got out the regulations, they said Guide Dogs for the Blind. "I'd write to the disabled officer for London Transport," he said, and gave me the address.

I didn't mind paying for Skipper, but it would be nice for pensioners with Hearing Dogs to be able to benefit from free travel on the buses and underground and also to be able to sit downstairs with their dogs. So I wrote to the disabled officer explaining this. A few weeks later I received a friendly interim reply saying that he was talking to Hearing Dogs, and the outcome is that now not only Skipper and other Hearing Dogs but all dogs enjoy free travel on London Transport. I hope other regions will follow London's example.

After the Heineken presentations life calmed down for a while in Subtitling and Skipper and I could retreat into obscurity. This was not to last for long, however. I had been subtitling *Blazing Saddles*, which was to be broadcast as part of a Mel Brooks season. In the film there is a notorious baked-bean scene, where the baddies consume loads of baked beans and emit lots of flatulent noises in typical Mel Brooks' style. I faithfully set about subtitling these low noises. "FRUUUURRPP!" I keyed every time one of them came up. After much fruuuurrp-ping, I began to wonder. I knew what was going on because it was in the script, but would the deaf know what these phonetic renderings were? After much debate and discussion with the other subtitlers, I decided to slip in a subtitle: "The farting continues", just to make sure that the deaf viewers had got the joke. I wondered about putting "flatulence", but that sounds a little too high-flown for Mel Brooks, so I decided to stick with "farting".

No sooner had *Blazing Saddles* been broadcast, than Mrs Mary Whitehouse was on the war-path. Evidently, a parent of a deaf child who was allowed to watch the programme at the late hour it was shown had been offended by the subtitling of the obscene noises, and had complained to Mrs Whitehouse. What amazed me was that this parent had not been offended by the bad language that had been very evident throughout the film, but had only switched off the set after the baked-bean scene, which was very near the end anyway. Mrs Whitehouse took up the cause. The deaf had to be protected from obscene noises that hearing people were allowed to hear!

Alan Rusbridger of *The Guardian* Diary reported this incident with great amusement and the deaf magazines, who took the matter more seriously than *The Guardian*, were outraged. "The deaf are normal people, not children, and don't need to be protected or patronised," deaf people wrote in an attempt to combat Mary Whitehouse's campaign to get Ceefax and Oracle sub-titling services under the Obscene Publications Act. Luckily, Mrs Whitehouse quietly allowed her outcry to die down, and subtitles remain a faithful rendering of the soundtrack of television programmes – and long may they remain so!

# 6

# Thank you, Loughborough

Not long after our first meeting at the *SuperStore* reception, Stella Binns invited Skipper and me to spend a weekend with her and Mike in Loughborough. This would be a great chance to say thank you to all the people who had helped Stella raise so much of the money for Skipper. We accepted by return of post.

I arranged to leave work early that Friday, hoping to beat the rush-hour traffic. However, a lot of other drivers had similar ideas, and getting to the M1 was a lengthy business. Skipper had noticed our weekend suitcase in the car and he sat expectantly on the front seat, looking out of the window and wondering where he was going. But, like many people, he soon got bored with the London traffic jams and smells, curled up and went to sleep, as if to say, wake me up when we get to wherever we're going.

It was raining heavily and I had my windscreen wipers on at full speed. Suddenly, halfway down the motorway to Loughborough, the wiper on the driver's side became very loose and stopped working. As I couldn't see where I was going I pulled over onto the hard shoulder. Breaking down on the motorway was something I had always dreaded and now it had actually happened. It was pouring so hard it looked as if the rain would never stop. And it was obvious that I couldn't go any further without my windscreen wipers. But how was I going to phone for help?

Leaving Skipper in the car I walked to the nearest phone box. I picked up the receiver and repeated that I was deaf, my AA number and the fact that I'd broken down, about ten times. Then I returned to the car, leaving the receiver off the hook and hoping that, if nobody had managed to get my message, someone would wonder why the receiver had been left hanging and come and investigate.

Skipper knew that something was wrong and he sat on my knee as if to say, don't worry. I'm here.

After about ten minutes, when I was beginning to give up hope, a police car drove up. "Can you understand us, or shall we write it down for you?" they asked.

I explained that I could understand them very well if they spoke clearly and slowly and faced me. They looked relieved, and I explained the problem, apologising for leaving the phone off the hook.

"Oh, don't worry about that," they replied. "That was exactly the right thing to do. That way we were able to locate you very quickly."

As they were unable to mend my wiper themselves, they radioed the AA who arrived ten minutes later. When I've broken down with friends, I've never known the AA to arrive so quickly, especially if there's a lot of holiday traffic around, so leaving the phone off the hook and getting the police was definitely the right thing to do!

We reached Loughborough without further mishaps. Skipper recognised Stella and Mike immediately and soon had them organised into playing games with him in their back garden.

This was the first of several happy visits to Stella and Mike. We travelled around Loughborough in the trusty blue Mini which had been so often piled to the rear window with goods for the countless rummage sales, summer fêtes, cheese and wine parties and coffee mornings that had contributed to the training of Skipper. As we went, I learnt how Stella had first heard about the Hearing Dogs people from her daughter Joy who taught the deaf. At one car-boot sale, someone had even tried to buy the Mini! Stella, along with her son Richard and her friends Moya, Audrey and Wynn, had been quite tireless and, despite finding that charity organisers had sometimes labelled their table "Hearing Dogs for the

Blind" or "Hearing-Aids for Dogs", the marathon fund-raising went on. I found it so difficult to convey my immeasurable gratitude adequately to the people of Loughborough. But Skipper, as usual, had no trouble at all, and entered into a licking marathon. Mum and dad also enjoyed meeting Stella and Mike. It wasn't long before we all felt we had known each other for ever.

With Stella I once attended a local British Association for the Hard-of-Hearing dinner-dance, but was really depressed by the sort of questions some people asked. Someone came up to Stella and said, "Does she drive? Does she talk?" These questions were a sad reminder of the schism that exists between deaf and hard-of-hearing people. The term "hard-of-hearing" is usually applied to those who develop a slight or severe hearing loss later on in life. The term "deaf" is either used for people who are born with a hearing defect or develop one when they are young. Some people who suffer from a slight hearing loss are very reluctant to enter a deaf world, a world they associate with silence, disability and sign language. The lack of integration between the two groups of people has led to many sad misunderstandings.

This is something which constantly upsets me. As far as I am concerned, however great the hearing loss, and however that hearing loss was acquired, we all suffer from the same problem. The sooner that deaf people, deafened and hard-of-hearing people get together to discuss their mutual problems the better. After all, the non hearing-impaired public can never be expected to understand our problems fully if we are not prepared to try and understand each other.

Meeting Stella and the people who had helped to raise the money for Skipper made me wish that I could fund-raise for Hearing Dogs, but my job was demanding and I didn't really have the time. "Don't worry," Stella advised me, "you're good publicity." What Stella said made sense. Not many deaf people enjoy appearing on television because they worry about how they will understand the interviewer and how their speech will be, as well as how their dog will perform in a distracting studio. Skipper and I did not face these problems to the same degree, because the studios were our place of work – so next time I met Gillian Lacey, I offered to help publicise Hearing Dogs this way.

It was not long before I was taken up on my offer rather more alarmingly than I'd bargained for. Gillian rang me at work. "Do you speak French?" she asked. I apologetically explained that I had opted out of modern languages at school. "But I saw some of your subtitles which were in very good French, so I thought you must speak it."

"Ruth and Elizabeth have both lived and studied in France," I explained. "When we want French subtitling, we ask them. All I do is the Latin." At Battle Abbey they had been quite happy for me to learn Latin as a reading language and never have to utter a word of it.

"Then perhaps you can help us between you?" Gillian continued hopefully. "There is somebody called Gabrielle starting up a Hearing Dogs association in Switzerland, and she wants someone to interview on the radio to tell people what the dogs do. I'm sure you can cope with that somehow, can't you?" Gillian gave me Gabrielle's number and I consulted Elizabeth.

"Here's what we'll do," said my resourceful colleague. "I'll talk to her in French first, and tell you what she wants, then hand over to you and mouth her words for you if she speaks enough English. Right, here goes."

Elizabeth dialled the number. Gabrielle's English was all right and soon I had plunged into telling her what Skipper meant to my sense of personal independence and confidence. "Gabrielle says that's wonderful," said Elizabeth, who had skilfully put all this into French as well, just to make sure. "And she wants me to add something." Elizabeth had no difficulty thinking what to say. "Skipper's a well-behaved little dog, who causes no problems in the office. He's so good-natured, and we love him dearly," she told Gabrielle, and Skipper, who had been watching us intently, seemed pleased with his good report.

A large parcel of truffles and some note-paper soon arrived for us from Gabrielle, together with a long letter about *Les Chiens pour Sourds* which she was founding. The first puppy she was training was appropriately named Chinnor after the British Centre. Not long afterwards, Skipper and I met Gabrielle when we visited the Hearing Dogs stand at Cruft's. Gabrielle had come over specially, and I invited her and all the other helpers on the stand to dinner.

Gabrielle was delighted to come and meet Skipper and see him at work. We made sure that she would be the first to arrive so she could see him answer the door for everyone else. I made sure that lots of people rang us and made lots of kettles boil. Skipper was rushed off his paws and Gabrielle was full of admiration for him. "It is not only the work that he does so well," she told me, "it is also the way that he always looks at you. It will be one thing to train a dog to do things, but to train a dog to have the relationship that you have! Is there anything you wish he could do for you which he does not do?"

"The only thing I wish he could do is tell me the bits I don't pick up in meetings at work," I joked.

"He tries," Gabrielle assured me. "He doesn't bark much, but he does make whimpers and sighs, and he greeted everyone with a different bark. He's the most human dog that I have met!"

One day, when I was subtitling *Dallas*, which had to be finished for the next day, my hearing-aid broke down. Without it I couldn't hear a thing, so was unable to use my special amplifier, and as I don't know if anything is being said off screen without it, I had to stop working. Not only was I unable to subtitle without my hearing-aid, I also could not use my telephone amplifier. So I had no way of checking that all was well before a programme went out that night.

I had no choice but to rush straight to the hospital and hope that they had a spare hearing-aid. As there were workmen in the office, I decided to take Skipper with me. At first the hospital receptionist was not too keen on Skipper, so I had to explain that he was a Hearing Dog who came to work with me. As my hearing-aid had broken down at work, I had nowhere to leave him and had to bring him with me to the hospital.

"Well, why can't you tie him up to the railings?" she asked. I was certainly not going to leave Skipper tied to a railing, and it was only when I asked her if she'd care to stand with Skipper, who was worth £2,500, that she relented and let me take him into the hospital.

But persuading her to let Skipper in was a minor problem compared with trying to get my hearing-aid repaired and borrow a spare one. The technician took one look at my Phonac aid, a high-powered private aid, given me on the NHS because NHS hearing-aids are not powerful enough to help me, and shrugged. "I can only replace NHS hearing-aids. You'll have to take that one to Rehabilitation. They deal with the private stuff." I found I had to make an appointment to see Rehabilitation, and there was not a spare appointment for two weeks. I had to finish *Dallas* by the next day!

I explained the situation, but nobody could or would help. I could not even leave the broken aid to be repaired until I had an appointment. If I had to wait two weeks to get an appointment, a further two or three weeks for the aid to be repaired, with no guarantee of getting a spare one, it looked as if I'd be without a hearing-aid and unable to work for a month. The prospect was daunting. Blistering with anger, I marched out of the hospital.

Ear, Nose and Throat hospitals have always made me feel deaf and disabled. I remember dreading visits to them as a small child – the endless sitting, queuing in corridors. Why were the other children in my class not there too? What had I done wrong? Then the long, drawn-out audiology tests with the heavy earphones weighing me down as I reacted to various pitches of bleeps by moving a toy brick. Even today I can't stand headphones because they remind me of that childhood torture.

I particularly remember one nightmare incident when I was seven. One night after school I blacked out. My grandparents panicked and called an ambulance. I was rushed off to a strange hospital with no ENT department. When my poor mother, who had been working that evening, was eventually contacted and arrived at the hospital, she was not allowed to see me. The sister on duty gave her a long lecture on how to look after her child, and sent her away. Because of the panic and because my mother was not allowed to see me, the hospital did not know that I was deaf. The next day they carried out a number of tests, thinking I was epileptic. Instead of headphones, wires were attached to my head. My family was not there and I was terrified. On top of this, I even got the usual audiology test, and I think it was then that I suddenly realised why I had to have the tests. All this time my ears were hurting very badly.

Eventually my mother was allowed to see me, and fortunately she had been round to our local GP, who was a friend of the family. He realised why I had blacked out. Many deaf people have inner-ear or middle-ear infections which cause them to lose their balance and pass out. Very little is known about how this happens, although I sometimes connect these recurrent infections with stress. When the hospital found this out, I was sent home with antibiotics.

Now, not being able to do my work because the hospital would not see me, or even take my aid to be repaired for two weeks, was the final straw. I was worried about finishing *Dallas* and felt helpless and angry. I was also wondering what another deaf person would do. If deaf people have to wait a month for a hearing-aid to be repaired and are not able to do any work in the meantime, it would certainly not encourage an employer to give them jobs.

When I got back to work, everyone was shocked. My boss rang the hospital but had no luck. Even the BBC doctor tried. Suddenly, one of the deaf people working in the subtitling unit had an idea. "Phone up the Royal National Institute for the Deaf. They might be able to help," she suggested. As I couldn't even phone the Royal National Institute for the Deaf without my hearing-aid, someone had to do it for me. Luckily, the RNID thought they might have a spare aid for me, so I raced round there.

The RNID didn't mind Skipper coming with me, and they had a spare Phonac aid which they said I could borrow, since it was in a good cause. I was so relieved. There would now be subtitles for the episode of *Dallas* when Bobby Ewing got shot!

"How come you have spare hearing-aids?" I asked the helpful technician.

"We don't really keep them as spares," she explained. "They are for sale. We encourage people to send us private aids which are no longer any use to them and then we service and sell them." I was just very lucky that they had a spare Phonac hearing-aid.

I was still angry with the hospital, and determined that no deaf person should suffer as I did. After all, it was the hospital's responsibility, not the RNID's, to provide me with a spare hearing-aid. And if I had been in a wheel-chair and my chair had broken, I was sure that they would not have left me stranded. So I wrote to the hospital and complained.

My letter certainly had an effect on the hospital! I did not tell them about the aid the RNID had lent me, as I wanted to get a spare one from the hospital so I could return the aid to the RNID as soon as possible, in case they wanted to sell it. So, when my hospital appointment came up two weeks later, I went along determined to do battle.

When I arrived at the hospital, with Skipper as a matter of principle, nobody questioned his presence. Instead of going to Rehabilitation, I was sent to see the specialist himself. He was very sorry about the whole affair and anxious to make amends. My broken hearing-aid was instantly repaired by an excellent technician and the specialist told me to get in contact with him if I ever had any problems again. I was relieved that this particular hospital nightmare was over. But still I wondered if another deaf person would have been so lucky. If ENT departments were not so short-staffed because of cutbacks, and if there were not a shortage of money to provide high-powered hearing-aids on the NHS, then deaf people would receive a better service from the hospitals.

7

## Songs of Praise

Skipper had been with me for a year and we were working so well together, both at home and at work. He seemed to have settled in to his routine and was always anxious to learn new ways of helping me. One day, when we were about to cross the road in Shepherd's Bush, he sat at the kerb and looked right and then left and right again. I saw a mother with two young children pointing to him, and soon the children were copying Skipper, looking carefully to the right and to the left. "Clever dog. You listen and I'll look," I told him. What Skipper would do if I crossed the road not having seen a car coming round the bend, I have still to find out, but we now have this routine when we are on our own.

In the office, Skipper was accepted and always very well behaved. Whilst I subtitled, he would lie patiently in his basket, only leaving it to alert me of a sound. He had given me so much confidence that I began to think of leaving Subtitling. I was deaf; I was working with people who understood deaf people and often wanted to discuss deafness because our subtitling was for the deaf. I was very aware of being deaf and I wondered how I would cope working in a part of the BBC that had nothing to do with the deaf. Could I manage? Deep down inside, I wanted to try and I wanted to feel that I was a person, not a deaf person. I felt I would have more chance of doing this if I was not having to think of deafness twenty-four hours a day.

At first I put these thoughts to one side, thinking that I would be deserting the hearing-impaired. "You mustn't think like that," a deaf friend told me. "You must go on in the BBC and do what you want to do. Of course you're not deserting us; you're proving what can be done." That made sense, and as we now had two more hearing-impaired subtitlers, I felt less bound to subtitling.

I had very little trouble in thinking of where I wanted to go. I wanted to work in Religious Programmes for a number of reasons. I had often subtitled *Songs of Praise* and was always moved when the people interviewed in the programme talked about how they had overcome a disability or problem, and the idea of working with members of the public who had never seen a camera, yet had something real to say that might help others, was a challenge.

I had also been interested in religion ever since I was at Battle Abbey. The girls at the Abbey came from a number of different religious backgrounds; there were Moslems, Hindus, Buddhists, Sikhs and Jews as well as Christians at the school. We all got on well and even discussed our different beliefs and incorporated them into our classes and assemblies. We never felt that some of us were right and the rest of us wrong. I was so fascinated by the different beliefs that I would try a different one for a week or month at a time. "I want to be a Hindu," I informed Bina, my Hindu friend. "I'd like to do everything that you do and you must explain what you believe in to me." Bina did, and among other things, I went without meat for the rest of the term.

Because of this interest, I always did very well in Religious Studies, even if I questioned everything. "There can't be a God of Love if people are hungry, disabled and suffer," I'd always argue. Deep down I suppose I wanted to know why I had to be deaf, and it took me many, many years to realise that having a problem like deafness makes life more challenging and makes you more aware and sensitive to other people's problems. Looking back, I now think that my life would have been meaningless if I had not had to overcome my deafness.

I confided my plans to Ruth, who thought that it was a good idea to apply for a job in Religion next time one was advertised. "But when they ask you why you want to work there, what are you going to say? You're not exactly God-squad," she asked curiously.

"Well, religious programmes are about people, and I am interested in the way that many people have had to cope with a number of things and I am interested in theology."

"All right," said Ruth, not entirely convinced of my motives. "Why did you study theology at university?"

"That was an accident," I replied and proceeded to tell Ruth what happened.

I had always got good grades in RE because of my questioning attitude, and kept it on to Scholarship-level because it seemed an easy exam to take. I hoped to go to Cambridge, and wanted to spend a year after my A-levels and S-levels taking the Oxbridge exam. My teachers were enthusiastic about my plans, and it came as a great shock to us all when I did not do so well in my A-level exams – except in RE, where I got the top grade. But this alone would not get me into Cambridge, and as all my hopes had been pinned on going there, I hadn't applied to any other university. "What are you going to do?" asked my mother, trying to break through my shock and depression.

Suddenly an idea came to me. "I'm going to drive round the country and turn up at every university until one takes me to do Law or anything. Can I borrow the car for a week?" I asked.

"I'll come and give you moral support," mum offered. We then packed our suitcases, leaving my shocked father to reason out if we had done the right thing.

"Where are we going first?" mum asked.

"Bristol," I replied. "I liked the look of the brochure."

We arrived at Bristol a few days before the term started and I went straight to the Senate House, leaving mum in the car. I explained my situation to the admissions officer in the Senate House, who was surprised, and not too pleased to see me! "You'll have to try and get in to a university through clearing, and you have left it too late for that," he told me. "And we don't take people with your grades anyway," he ended.

I was very depressed. I felt rejected and I had to tell my poor mother who had been dragged away on a wild-goose chase what had happened. As I came out of the Senate House I saw some beautiful gardens and decided to have a quiet cry there before telling her the news. In this park was a beautiful Regency building with "Theology Department" on the door. I don't know what prompted me, but I did a crazy thing. I went in to the department to the reception. "I've just been to the Senate House and they suggested that I see the admissions tutor here," I informed the receptionist, wincing at the lie. The receptionist looked surprised, but told me to wait, and it was not long before I was taken to see Dr Gill, the admissions tutor, who was even more surprised to see me.

I decided to tell him the truth: that the Senate House hadn't sent me and that I was desperate. "Not everyone gets an S-level grade one," he told me, "and it doesn't make sense that you should get that result and then the others. Can I contact your teachers?" I gave him the number of the school and some names and he went away to phone. "Your teachers are as surprised as you are about your results," he told me on his return. "Let's discuss your papers."

We discussed my A-level courses and the subjects I had studied for what seemed an age. "Congratulations," Dr Gill informed me after he had finished, "you've earned yourself a place. Term starts in a week and I expect to see you here. Fill in these forms and I'll find you a place in a hall of residence."

It was such a relief to go to university after all, that I did not have enough time to think about how I would follow in lectures. Dr Gill had not seen any problems. "Do a lot of reading, borrow lecture notes, and I'm sure that the lecturers will be only too pleased to explain things to you," was all he had to say when I told him that I was deaf. He was right. The lecturers took care to write all the difficult words on the blackboard, and were always happy to spend an hour or so explaining anything that I did not understand. I read as much as I could to make up for what I did not hear in lectures and discussed this with them.

Seminars I found difficult. Following confident lecturers who faced me was one thing; trying to understand nervous students mumbling desperately in seminars was another. My Philosophy of Religion lecturer had the answer. "Don't take subjects where there are bound to be large seminars. Take courses with small seminar groups of about four or five. Don't choose your subjects until everyone else has chosen." This was sound advice.

I was determined to make a real effort to integrate and get involved with university life, and not to spend all my time studying. I had no problems doing this. It was the first year that girls had been admitted into the hall of residence that I was in, and we were a very small minority there. It came as a surprise when I found on my second day that I had been nominated to run the hall sports. What came as a worse surprise was learning that I would have to make a speech and answer questions from the floor in connection with this. I felt really sick! Nevertheless I decided to be cool, and with a great effort said my speech and then explained that I was deaf. Could anyone who wanted to ask questions address the chairman, who, I hoped, would repeat the question to me. Everyone clapped, no one asked any questions, and I was duly elected.

Running the hall sports led to other things and soon I was involved in the University Entertainments and countless clubs. "Why don't you stand for Vice-President of the Union?" my friend Nick suggested during my last year. Being Vice-President would mean a year running student activities paid for by the Students' Union. I wouldn't have to look for a job straight away and it would be fun and worthwhile. The more I thought about Nick's suggestion, the more enthusiastic I became. The following year was to be the International Year of the Disabled and as Vice-President I could really push the university to accept more disabled students and do something about helping them when they got there. At the time there was no wheel-chair access at Bristol, while I myself would have been enormously helped if they had installed a portoscribe in the lecture halls. This is a gadget that allows notes to be projected on a screen or a wall. It's one thing to be promised a loan of a friend's lecture notes, quite another to decipher their private hieroglyphics, and near exam time nobody's too keen on parting with notes anyway. I had had to struggle, and my lecturers had helped me a lot. So I had all sorts of ideas I wanted to put into practice. I decided to stand.

"But what party shall I stand for?" I asked Nick. Bristol ran its elections on party political lines and I had always been apolitical.

"Well then, stand as an Independent, if that's what you are." Several of my friends stood for various offices as Independents too. It was going to be hard work, because Bristol was a university with a strong Liberal tradition. However, I decided to enjoy the campaign and Nick and another friend, Carol, agreed to help with publicity.

Night after night Vince, who was standing for Treasurer as an Independent, and I trudged round hall after hall, department after department, canvassing and putting up posters. When they could, Nick and Carol came too. Nick and another friend Curtis borrowed a long ladder and placed my posters out of reach from my opponents, who might tear them down. In fact, some are still there today because they are so unreachable! At this stage, we were all enjoying ourselves. Then came the hustings. As luck would have it, the first meeting was in the hall of residence that the Liberal candidate came from and this meant that the hall would be behind him. I was also worried because I would have to make a speech and answer questions from the floor in a strange hall and from people who might not know me. Nick was unable to go, but Carol and Vince would be there. "We'll take notes during your opponents' speeches and tell you what people ask you," they promised.

Thanks to their notes, I was able to take advantage of my opponents' weaknesses and attack them in my speech, but half way through I became aware of Carol making signs that I was to speak louder. I was sure that I was speaking as loud as I could. I knew something was wrong and began to lose confidence. "A bunch of Liberals were making a noise at the back, and you couldn't hear them, but they drowned most of what you said," Carol explained. "If only you'd heard them, you could have told them to shut up." I felt sick and miserable, especially as I was going to have to answer questions from the floor when the other candidates had finished speaking.

When question time started Carol came up on the platform with me to tell me what the questions were. "That's not allowed," said one Liberal, and a row developed over procedure, accompanied by loud shouts from the Liberals in the audience.

"I'll answer questions without Carol then," I insisted, desperate to avoid a scene. But I was upset and made a mess of question time – a truly inglorious beginning, I thought, and this is only the first session.

I was beginning to think of withdrawing, when the Socialist Worker and Tory chairmen came up to me. "What happened was disgusting. They knew you couldn't hear their shouting and that's why they did it, and they also knew that preventing Carol from helping you with questions would hamper you. Don't worry, we'll see it doesn't happen again and, if it's any consolation, you have our second votes." This really cheered me up. In a system where there are several rounds of voting and people vote for candidates in order of preference, to have the support of the extreme left and right would help me to combat the Liberals in the middle if I survived the first round.

This made me a little more confident for the next confrontation. Nick, Carol and Vince took notes for me again and when it was my turn to speak, the person chairing the meeting ordered absolute silence in the hall and during questions, Nick was allowed to write them down for me. Things were looking up, and my main problem now was convincing potential voters that I was truly independent of party, and not politically naive.

It was a hard-fought campaign and really opened my eyes to politics. I never expected the back-biting and bitter competition that developed. "I don't make promises I can't fulfil," I told people, and made a few practical promises. My opponent promised everything, and with the strong Liberal majority he was eventually elected. But I had learnt and experienced a great deal.

To apply for a job in a department of the BBC that was unaware of the problems of the deaf required a bit of courage, but the memory of standing in that election at Bristol convinced me that I could weather the board and possible rejection. I had to wait for a few months before an advertisement for a temporary job in Religious Programmes appeared in *Ariel*, the BBC's internal magazine.

"You don't stand a chance of getting that," my colleagues in Subtitling warned me as I applied for an assistant producer's job. "You've absolutely no experience of filming or anything."

But I was undaunted. "No harm in trying," I told them, "and even if I don't get it, I might get a board, which will be good practice, and if I don't get that, there's nothing lost."

"Well, so long as you don't get upset if you *don't* even get a board," said Ruth, worried.

I didn't honestly expect a board and was very surprised when I did get one. "There's no way I can get this job," I thought, "so I'll just enjoy myself and put in some board-attending practice." I decided not to take Skipper. Somebody might not like dogs. I'd cross that bridge when I came to it. But when I arrived at the board everyone asked where Skipper was and seemed disappointed that he had not come. All his scene-stealing over the past year had created him a fan club! This broke the ice and the interview went well. All good experience, I thought.

But I was in for a real surprise! David Wilson, the

Teletext manager, came to see me. "It looks like you're going to be leaving us," he began. My heart sank; was I about to be fired or made redundant? "Religious Programmes are not going to give you the job you applied for," he continued, confirming my worst fears, "but they are going to give you a six-month attachment as a researcher. You start in September."

I couldn't believe it! "But I only applied for the job for board practice."

"It looks like you have got a little more than that."

Once I had got over the excitement of going to Religious Programmes, I began to panic. Would anyone help me on the telephone? Would I get patronised or just left to do what I could? Would Skipper be accepted there?

"Think positively," Ruth advised. "If they thought you couldn't do the job, they wouldn't have given it to you; and they know all about Skipper. What we have to do is to make sure that you can use a phone independently."

The personnel officer, was very helpful. "Take one of the special amplified phones from Subtitling. That will save waiting around to have one fitted in *Songs of Praise*."

Perhaps I should try and explain about my phones. The specially amplified phone with its black vibrator was fine for the limited use I made of it in Subtitling, where most calls were an entirely predictable checking on technical hitches with familiar technicians' voices at the other end, saying what I expected to hear. But for initiating more general conversations, making appointments, taking down names and addresses and train times from strangers, this phone was not good enough. An additional earpiece was attached to my phone through which a colleague can listen in and mouth the other half of the conversation for me to lip-read. This has the virtue of being simple and almost simultaneous, but of course it does rely on someone else's goodwill.

Before going to *Songs of Praise* I was desperate to find a system that would allow me to be in total control on the telephone. Then I remembered reading in *No Need to Shout* about a new RNID telephone-bureau scheme. This This involves a three-way conversation, requiring Tandata keyboard equipment. The bureau operator keys the other party's conversation, which appears on a monitor screen for the deaf person, who can either speak in reply, as I do, or type back a response if they have a speech problem. It seemed the answer to all my self-sufficiency worries. "Get one," said David, when I explained it to him.

One day, the phone rang. "Hello," said a cheerful voice. "I'm Leila, and I hear that you're coming to us for six months on *Songs of Praise*. I'm a researcher too and perhaps we could have lunch so that I can tell you what you'll be doing. If I meet you in Ceefax I'll recognise Skipper."

What would I say to her? Meeting new people was still a bit of an ordeal. Leila was having much the same worries about me. Stephen Whittle, the editor of *Songs of Praise*, had suggested we have lunch and poor Leila wondered how she would manage to communicate with me. In fact, we got on immediately and had a lot in common, and the two-hour lunch had gone before we realised that we were meant to be discussing *Songs of Praise*.

"What you'll be doing is great fun and very straight forward," Leila explained. "When we decide that we are doing a *Songs of Praise* from say . . . Norwich, you go to Norwich and meet as many members of the congregations as you can to build up a picture of the communities there. You find out about the cultural history and anything that you think is of interest. You also have to find and recommend the people that we interview in the programme." That seemed to be more or less what I had expected to be doing, but one thing was still unanswered.

"How much will I have to use the telephone?" I asked, explaining my fears to Leila.

"Well, you will have to use the phone a lot, but don't worry, I'll be around to help you and we're not an uncaring bunch of people. Someone will always bail you out when you get stuck on the phone, I'm sure." This went a long way towards putting my worries at rest, and if everyone there was like Leila, it was going to be all right.

Leila paused. "I hope that you don't mind me asking, but I'm really curious. How will you cope with music? Can you hear it or don't you bother with it? I mean, if someone asks for a particular hymn or tune, will you know what they're talking about?"

I explained that music has great potential for deaf people as it covers a vast range of frequencies, from very high to very low notes, and there's often something in music that most deaf people can detect. Besides, even if they can't hear anything, there's so much vibration that it's very difficult to feel cut off from music, even if you are deaf. I explained that James, a musical friend of mine, had even tried to teach me to sing. He taught me to feel different notes in my throat and to remember which feeling corresponded to which note on a musical scale. I don't always hit the right note, but at least I don't sing flat any more and I try and restrict my singing to the bathroom. I explained to Leila that these lessons had helped me to subtitle *Songs of Praise*. I'd look at the music and count how many seconds in a line and check that the congregation were singing the hymn to that speed by vibration and hearing a bit, then put in the subtitles with the timing right. Usually I can even tell which tune a hymn is played to and recognise hymns by feeling the tune.

I left the canteen feeling a lot more optimistic about leaving Subtitling. If everybody was as helpful and as interested as Leila had been, I was sure that I would have no problems at *Songs of Praise*.

8

# First Assignment

I had been counting the days until I started in Religious Programmes and now the day had come. I had spent a sleepless night. I was scared stiff. All the old worries about communicating with new people churned round and round inside me, despite my happy encounter with Leila. I resisted the urge to take the day off sick and drove into Television Centre. I resisted the urge, then, to go back to the Subtitling Unit, and Skipper gave me a surprised "is this right?" look when, instead of walking into the main building, we turned left into East Tower. The fact that I was staggering under his basket, my amplified telephone, my RNID phone, and his bones and toys, nearly dropping all of them, did not seem to upset Skipper. But he knew we were going somewhere new.

Everyone in *Songs of Praise* was very welcoming, but I was still fighting the urge to run all the way back to the Subtitling Unit.

"Your first programme," said Stephen, "is the Remembrance programme. It's coming from Newcastle Cathedral, and since so many of the North Eastern regiments fought in the Far East during the Second World War, the programme will feature the Far Eastern War. Valetta will help you and go with you to Newcastle."

I must have gone a paler shade of white when I heard all this. Geordie accents would be jumping in at the deep end. And Remembrance! What a programme to start on! I was hoping for a nice rural programme to find my feet in. The last Remembrance programme, I rapidly remembered, had come from Portsmouth and the Normandy beaches and it had been unbeatable.

Things seemed to get worse as Stephen continued, "The theme will be reconciliation." I swallowed. I knew a little bit about Japanese culture and a little bit about the war in the Far East, and I knew how bitter some of the men still were who had fought there and suffered unspeakable cruelties in prisoner of war camps. On the other hand, what about Japanese feelings over the atomic bombing of Hiroshima and Nagasaki? What a programme to have to start on! But what a challenge!

"Here's the file," said Stephen.

I hoped I managed to sound confident as I said, "I'll get on with it then." I went and asked Valetta what I should do as I had no idea what the procedure was, wishing that Leila was not away filming.

"I'm very busy with Rothwell," she said, "but if you'll set up some appointments for the end of the week, I'll come up to Newcastle with you." It was unbelievable. Nobody was holding my hand or being patronising. Quite the other extreme! I was being treated like any other new recruit: sink or swim. Well, I certainly wasn't going to sink.

I went through the names in the file. The clergy had put forward very few names of people who had fought in the war, let alone in the Far East. The Burma Star Association and the Far Eastern Prisoners of War had proposed a few people, however, and that was a start. I sat and stared at the phone and worried about Geordie accents and then gingerly picked it up, looking around me. I put it back down again. A few minutes later, I did the same thing. I couldn't summon up the courage to ring anybody.

"Do you want any help?" asked one of the production assistants called Sally. "I'm not very busy and if you need a hand with telephone calls I'd be only too pleased to help." I was very relieved and between us we made several calls. But we still needed more people. How was

I going to find people who had fought in the Far East?
I sat down and thought.

Then I remembered subtitling *Tenko*, the television
series about women in prison camps in the Far East. I
went round to see Ken Riddington, the producer. He
wasn't in, but his assistant was very helpful. "Oh, you
must get in touch with Anne Valery, who was our
adviser on *Tenko*," she said. "She knows hundreds of
women who were in the Far East and she'll be able to
put you in touch with the right people. And the other
place that was very helpful was the Imperial War
Museum. You ought to go down and see them."

This cheered me up. I soon had a long list of names
from Anne Valery and that afternoon I went round to
the Imperial War Museum, who put me in touch with a
university professor at Durham, who had written a book
called *Burma: the Longest War;* he in his turn put me in
touch with more people. The snowball had really got
going. And whenever I got stuck with phone calls, there
was Sally, always willing to help.

Finally, the end of the week came round and it was
time for Valetta and me to go to Newcastle. Skipper had
been farmed out to a friend just for this first time I told
him, while I coped with meeting new people and driving
round an unknown town in a hired car.

Our first stop was Durham, where we had arranged
to pick up the hired car. The train arrived on time, but
there was no hired car. After searching every corner of
the station with a resigned look on her face, Valetta decided to ring BBC Transport. I was feeling very sick. What
would I do if this happened to me when I was on my
own? How on earth would I phone Transport? I began
to wonder whether I was doing the right job, whether I
shouldn't just go back to London and explain to Stephen
that there was no way I could continue. But I told myself
firmly that when the time came things would work out.

When Valetta had finished her phone call, I asked her
if this happened frequently.

"Oh yes, it does," was her less than comforting reply.
Evidently the car hire firm had been expecting us the

following day, and we had to wait while they brought us a car from Newcastle. As our first appointment was in five minutes' time, this was bad news. When the car eventually arrived, an hour later, the fact that it was a large Rover was very little consolation.

We started on our round of interviews an hour late, and it didn't help that there were several streets, not to mention villages, with the same name. We started off by going to the wrong Sunniside and it took us two hours to find the right Sunniside. It amazed me that day how, despite the fact that we were late everywhere, the people we visited were all so welcoming and willing to talk about their painful experiences. I learnt a lot from Valetta and only asked the occasional question. Bit by bit I began to feel more and more confident. I had expected people to make no allowance for my hearing loss but I was quite wrong. They were understanding and only too willing to help. If I didn't get something, they patiently repeated it.

Valetta and I returned to London pleased with the people we had found. "What happens next?" I asked.

Valetta explained that we reported back to Stephen, the editor, and Noel, the producer. Then between us we tried to pick people from as many different denominations as possible. It's no good having them all from one church. And in this case we also had to try and blend Army, Navy and Air Force memories.

After much discussion we decided that in the programme we would interview: the army officer who had tried so hard to forgive the Japanese for what they had done to him, but could never forgive them for what they had done to his men; the RAF man who was imprisoned in Java and suffered much hardship there, and who after the war had defended the dropping of the atomic bombs on Hiroshima and Nagasaki, until one day at Speaker's Corner he had challenged Donald Soper to a debate, lost, and completely changed his viewpoint, and now he campaigned regularly for CND. There was a nurse who had trained in Newcastle Royal Infirmary and nursed the forces, both POWs and Japanese in Rangoon;

and the clergyman who, despite the hard conditions in the camps, had done all he could to administer Communion and keep normal religious life going. And there was the welfare officer of the Far Eastern Prisoners of War Association, who cared for the prisoners of war when they returned home from the Far East, suffering from incurable diseases that would haunt them for the rest of their lives. He still goes round visiting them and their widows and spends many hours trying to persuade the Pension Board that the illnesses many of them are suffering now are the result of their war service.

We also mentioned the well-known Remembrance prayer that the members of the Far Eastern Prisoners of War Association and the Burma Star Association would like us to use as it is inscribed on the memorial to the thousands of men who fell at the Battles of Imphal and Kohima:

> When you go home, tell them of us and say:
> For your tomorrow we gave our today.
> At the going down of the sun and in the morning
> We will remember them.

There was also a strong feeling about the three-minute silence. Stephen and Noel agreed to have a one-minute silence in the programme as a mark of respect for those who fell in the wars.

Though they were pleased with what we had suggested, they felt that something was missing. "I think we must have a ship-builder in the programme," said Noel. Newcastle had indeed been a centre of ship-building during the war.

"You'll have to go back to Newcastle and find a ship-builder," Stephen told us. Valetta explained that she was far too busy with Rothwell. "Oh well," said Stephen, looking at me. "You'll have to go back on your own."

I had more visions of cars not turning up. And anyway, how was I going to find a ship-builder? If I remembered rightly, the ship-yards of both Swan Hunter and Wallsend were closed by a strike at the time.

Sally and I rang the Wallsend yard. "I'm terribly sorry, all the men are on strike," was the answer. "You can't speak to anyone."

We put the phone down, our hearts sinking. Then I had an idea. We rang the ship-yard back. "Oh hello," I said. "It's the BBC here. We're making a programme about Newcastle and would like to include the ship-yards."

The man who answered the phone must have thought I was from the *News*, because before we could say bingo, the shop steward was on the line. "Are you coming to cover our strike?" he asked in a very strong Geordie accent. But I couldn't give him a false impression and my resolve crumbled. I explained where I was from and that we were doing a *Songs of Praise* from Newcastle for Remembrance Sunday.

However, he turned out to be a regular *Songs of Praise* viewer, so was only too willing to help. "I'll put you in touch with some of the men who worked in the yard during the war," he promised. "Let me put you through to our archivist, I'm sure he worked here then, too."

The archivist and I made a date and Skipper and I set off on the train to Newcastle. Not wanting to risk any problems with a hired car, I got a taxi from the station to the ship-yard. But when I arrived, there was no picket line and nobody in the yard. Had I made a mistake about the date? No, Sally had written it down for me. I walked round the yard trying desperately to find someone, but as there was nobody there I waited patiently outside the office.

Eventually, a very cheerful lady came along. "Oh," she exclaimed. "Yes, we are expecting you, but there have been so many redundancies that this is the last day in the yard for many of the men. They're having their leaving lunch. They won't be long, I promise you."

Soon, three ship-builders arrived who had worked in the yard during the war. "There is only one way," they said, "to tell you about our experiences here in the war, and that is to take you round the yard."

I couldn't think of a better way to learn about their experiences. It wasn't long before they were blowing a whistle and a chauffeur-driven car arrived. "Hop in," they said, "and we'll tell you about the war."

It was one of the most moving days of my life. I saw the docks on the Tyne that once had berthed so many ships, that had supported the war effort and suffered heavy bombardment, now empty with no ships in berth. I met the Strike Committee, fighting relentlessly for the jobs that they had done – jobs that their fathers and grandfathers had done before them. I went round the memorials and the houses where the ship-builders live and I realised that I was visiting a dying community and felt very sad. But I knew I had found three ship-builders.

I went back to London feeling pleased with myself. But if I thought I was finished with the Remembrance programme I was mistaken.

"What we need now," Stephen said, "is some old war film to go on top of the commentary."

Where was I to find film? I decided to go back to the Imperial War Museum, who had been so helpful in suggesting people to us. "Oh, we've got lots of film of the Far Eastern War," they said, "or rather, we've got all there is of it. You're very welcome to come and look. But we must warn you that some of it is nitrate film."

"Oh, that doesn't matter," I replied blithely. "I'm sure I'll manage." I put the phone down and went to ask what was wrong with nitrate film. I learnt it was remarkably prone to explode and needed very careful handling.

"Don't worry," said Simon, one of my colleagues. "I used to be a film editor. Handling nitrate film isn't difficult. I'll come along and help you out."

What we saw at the Imperial War Museum was unbelievable. There was film of men in the prisoner of war camps, who no longer looked like men, undignified, grabbing cigarettes from their liberators. There was film of the Battles of Imphal and Kohima, film of people lying dead and dying in agony, in mud and mire, film of the humiliated Japanese trying to commit *hara-kiri*. There was film of the Japanese standing at Hiroshima and Nagasaki, staring at places where two proud towns had once stood. Much of this was unsuitable for *Songs of Praise*, but nevertheless we arranged to have it copied.

The only thing missing was some film of the Burma railway. Three of our interviewees had worked on the notorious Railway where so many thousand allied prisoners of war had died. I was mentioning this problem to Jennifer, one of my friends who worked in the News Film Library, and wondering if I would have to give up.

"I'm sure we've got some of that," she said, and to my amazement she discovered some film in the BBC Film Library. I had this copied without delay.

I now had all the film that we needed for the programme. It was a grand experience to see the film rushes of the interviews, and to learn that in an editing studio even the most stuttering and hesitant person can be made to seem eloquent. It was an even greater thrill to look in the *Radio Times* and see my name under the billing. My mother had a field day. She went out and bought hundreds of copies! All my friends were joking and saying that Skipper ought to have his credit too.

It was more moving to watch the programme. Even today, whenever I watch that programme I am moved. I hope that it led many people to remember the sufferings of those who fought in the Far East, who are known as "the forgotten army". At Wood Lane it was agreed that the Newcastle programme was every bit as good as the previous year's Remembrance programme. But to me what really mattered was that it might have opened the eyes of viewers who had never paid any attention to the Far Eastern war and stirred them to give some practical thought, maybe, to easing that war's legacy of pain and suffering still being experienced by its survivors today.

9

# The Mersey Sound

As researching the Christmas programme in Canterbury promised to be hectic, and Valetta would be with me, I decided to leave Skipper in London with my friend Olga. It was the first anniversary of Skipper coming to me, and for want of a more accurate date, his birthday. So I packed some chicken in his suitcase as a special birthday treat. But if I thought that Skipper was going to go without any birthday presents I was wrong! Olga's father gave him a pork pie, and as soon as David Kremer, one of the producers on *Songs of Praise*, heard that it was Skipper's birthday, a packet of custard creams arrived from the tea-bar.

During the time I was in Canterbury, Olga was due to attend a costing seminar in Elstree, where *EastEnders* is made, and, as Skipper has his own staff identity card, Olga assumed that there would be no problem in taking him with her. But when she drove into Elstree, the security man on the gate took one look at Skipper and said, "No dogs, miss."

"But he's a BBC dog. He's allowed in," Olga replied.

"Oh, so he's in a production! Is he an *EastEnder* dog, then?"

As Olga is not an avid *EastEnder* fan, she failed to grasp exactly what the security man meant. "He's not an *EastEnder*, he's a Westender," she answered, thinking he was referring to Skipper's place of abode.

"In that case, he can't come in." Olga had made many *Heart of the Matter* and *Everyman* programmes about different kinds of discrimination in society, but this was

0

the first she'd heard about discriminating against a dog because he came from the West End and not the East End of London, so she assumed that the security man was having her on. "OK, then, he's an East End dog, so let him in!"

"Look, no dogs, miss," was his final, unamused reply.

Luckily, I'd left Skipper's BBC identity card and his Hearing-Dog certificate with Olga, so she was able to produce them as evidence of Skipper's bona fides. But the display of these cards provoked a shattering change of attitude in the security man. All of a sudden he began to mouth words slowly and gesture. "OH . . . *I see.* Your dog CAN come in. You can park just there, near me, and I will help you."

Olga was speechless. One minute she was having a normal, joking conversation, the next being treated like an idiot. The sort of incident that deaf people take for granted was an eye-opener for her. And it was only after Olga had told me of this incident that I realised how much I had accepted a patronising attitude as normal.

Despite this inauspicious start, Skipper enjoyed the costing seminar. Everyone made a great fuss of him. Meanwhile, I was missing him horribly in Canterbury. During the day, Valetta and I were so busy doing our research that I hardly had time to miss him. But at night I became very insecure without him. How would I wake up in the morning, and how would I know if there was a fire in the hotel, I wondered.

Valetta was very reassuring. "If you don't come down to breakfast by eight thirty, I'll come and get you; and I've never stayed in a hotel where there was a fire." All the same I was pleased that my room was on the ground floor and I could easily jump out of the window.

Despite Valetta's promise to wake me if need be, I remembered a similar incident in my pre-Skipper days, when Alison from *No Need to Shout* and I were attending a British Deaf Association conference in Torquay. When I didn't appear at breakfast, Alison came to wake me and, of course, found that the door was locked. She tried knocking, with no success whatsoever. Luckily, I *was* awake and in the process of coming down to breakfast, so I discovered Alison on her way to find a spare key.

This was one of the incidents which had strengthened my resolve to apply for a Hearing Dog. Working in Ceefax did not involve many stays in hotels, but I knew that if I ever did get into production I would have to cope in a hotel on my own. Bells, fire-alarms, knocks on doors could happen in hotels. After feeling so insecure without Skipper in Canterbury, I resolved that I would never leave him behind again when I was working on location, even if I had one of my colleagues with me. So a battered and paw-trampled Skipper found himself accompanying me on the morning rush-hour tube to Euston, bound for Liverpool.

At least I already had my ticket. Booking train tickets face to face with someone you know in the BBC's travel office is a luxury for a deaf person. Getting a ticket at a railway station is very frustrating if you have to rely on lip-reading. The grids at the ticket desks are invariably not at eye level, and often besmirched with dirt, which makes it impossible to lip-read the ticket man behind them. Unless you speak through the grid he is unable to hear you, and unless you face him through the clear glass, not the grid, he cannot be lip-read.

As usual, the ticket inspector queried why Skipper hadn't got a ticket, and I was thankful that I had asked British Rail's officer for the disabled to give me a covering letter, explaining that Skipper travels free on trains because he is a Hearing Dog. The production of his certificate and orange lead and collar does not always convince a ticket collector of his status, but we were all right that day.

Once under way Skipper curled up on the floor beside me, until the buffet opened and our fellow passengers began sharing their breakfasts with him. By the time we reached Lime Street station, everyone in the compartment knew how to communicate with hearing-impaired people and what Hearing Dogs were!

The hotel I had arranged to stay in didn't mind dogs, especially after I had explained how Skipper would help me in the hotel. Normally they charged extra for animals, but in Skipper's case they waived this rule.

Skipper is a born traveller. He is seldom confused by new surroundings, especially if he has someone he knows with him. After an initial inspection, he soon settled down beside the radiator in the hotel room. And after what had proved to be an exhausting day, trying to find my way round Liverpool and talking to a number of young people, I was thankful that I could just go to sleep and not worry about oversleeping in the morning or the remoter possibility of a hotel fire.

November seems a funny month to be researching for Palm Sunday, but as cathedrals cost so much to light, it is not unusual to record two programmes at once, and a colleague was doing one for Epiphany at the same time. I was looking forward to researching ours, as it was to be a young people's programme. Finding young people who can talk well about their faith is always a challenge, and I really had to go hunting for mine because the schools were all shut and the teachers on strike. But the Liverpool clergy couldn't have been more enthusiastic and helpful. The university Catholic chaplain and the father in charge of youth work both jumped in their cars and within an hour had rounded up their young flock for me to meet. Teaching nuns forgot about the dispute for an hour as they collected some of their pupils for me. The Anglican and free churches also gave me lists of youngsters to call on.

The issue I came up against on every side, however, was unemployment. In Liverpool it was staggering. Most of the kids I met had families who were suffering the long-term hardships that unemployment brings, yet most were confident that they and Liverpool would emerge from their problems. The fact that many of their school or college courses were cancelled and they might not get their educational qualifications, and would leave school to go on the dole anyway, did not dampen their spirits. I wondered if the fact that they were Christians

93

was what accounted for their extraordinary optimism.

"We are the future of Liverpool," quite a few of them told me confidently.

"It's a beautiful city," one girl said, "and Liverpudlians are hardworking. All we need is for the rest of the country to realise this and have confidence to invest in us."

"Do you think that will happen?" I asked, knowing that both her parents had been unemployed for quite a long time.

"I'm sure it will," she replied.

Liverpool made me remember my own period of unemployment. I had graduated from Bristol confident that the world was my oyster, but I was soon to discover how useless an arts degree was without job experience. I decided not to mention I was deaf on job application forms. If and when I got an interview I would say that I had a *slight* hearing problem, but not before. I was lucky to be able to live at home with mum and dad and I repaid them by being bad tempered and apathetic, rousing myself on Monday to scour the arts and media pages of *The Guardian* and fill in endless application forms. I tried the local Job Centre briefly, too, though again I decided not to register as disabled.

"Do you have any jobs which are not in catering?" I'd ask the grumpy man in the half-rimmed glasses.

"Well, what experience do you have?" he'd mumble, looking at me over the top of them.

"Oh, I've got a degree in theology and I've done a lot of vacation jobs."

"Yes, but what *real* experience do you have?" Good question. After three months of this I became a waitress in a transport café. My deafness didn't bother the manageress and I was more than capable of taking orders. At worst I could ask people to point at the menu.

I still filled in job application forms and even got a few interviews with some local firms. Those early job interviews were a nightmare! When I arrived for my first with a local printing firm, I couldn't sum up the courage to go in, and stood on the doorstep wondering what I would tell mum and dad. I was so ashamed, I even lied to my parents, telling them that the interview had been a success. I could not do this again, so I turned up for my next interview with a local insurance firm, determined to do well. As I had difficulty understanding the interviewer, I said that I was a little hard of hearing and he began to speak more clearly. I did not get the job, but at least I was in the swing of interviews.

Then I heard that if you were unemployed for six months, you were eligible for Manpower Services Commission schemes that looked as if they were geared to giving graduates initial working experience to enable them to apply for management jobs. So I decided to leave the café and qualify for one of those schemes. Mum had worked out how I would fill in the six months of waiting to be eligible! She wanted me to improve my communication skills, and although my speech was now good, bar a slight lisp, my understanding of what strange people said could have been better. Mum contacted David Beeching, whose Adult Education lip-reading classes I tried to attend when I was at Battle Abbey, but then I had been under age.

David is not really a lip-reading teacher; he is a communication specialist. Lip-reading, as it is misleadingly termed, is not merely understanding what people say by watching lip-patterns. Lip-patterns on their own only amount to about sixty per cent of any conversation and it is the expression on the speaker's face and the possible subjects of conversation that help the lip-patterns to make sense. Really, lip-reading ought to be called face-reading. Everybody instinctively learns some of the skills of face-reading; some of us need to rely more on them than others. A person who is born deaf acquires a natural ability to lip-read, while somebody who goes deaf later on in life can find learning which lip-patterns make which sounds a real struggle.

Having gone deaf very early, my lip-reading was by no means poor, but David was able to develop my instinctive ability. I learnt what lip-shapes made what sounds, something I never before dwelt upon consciously. I also learnt which sounds could easily be confused. Who would think that eight and nine look alike when they are casually said? David taught me how to get around these problems. Instead of saying, "Did you say eight or nine?" to which the answer would invariably be either eight or nine, he taught me how to ask a closed question: how to say "Did you say nine?" so that the answer would be either "Yes" or "No". He also advised me on where to sit in order to follow conversations better. "Don't sit facing bright sunlight," he'd advise. "Sit with your back to the sunlight so that it does not get in your eyes and always sit in good light."

David's tuition also helped me to gain more confidence, and to make more use of the little residual hearing I had when wearing my phonic-ear hearing-aids. Recognising certain lip-patterns as "ooh" or "aah" was a start, and with a high-pitched speaker like mum, I can identify the odd consonant once in a while. Instead of just battling to make a conversation with somebody, I'd think more about what they were likely to be talking about, and even rapidly change the conversation if I got lost. My rather ungraceful "What? I didn't hear," became, "I'm sorry, I didn't catch what you said. Were you talking about your holiday?" A closed question, and one that didn't admit I had a hearing loss. David and mum explained that at parties, with all the noise going on, even hearing people can't always hear. So only when I got really stuck would I admit to being deaf. Now I think I'm better off than hearing people at parties. The background noise doesn't bother me and I carry on as normal.

David also gave me help with job interviews. He reassured me that interviewers usually use the information in the application form to guide them in their line of questioning, and he advised me on the best way to explain at the start of the interview about my deafness without putting the interviewer off. "Say to them: I do have a hearing loss, and I must see your faces when you talk. So if you don't all talk to me at once, I'd really appreciate it! But, don't worry, I'll understand you perfectly well if you do this."

Now I was prepared, I couldn't wait for my next job interview, but life is never what you expect, and my next interview came about in a most surprising way. One day, Rosalie, our next-door neighbour, came round waving a newspaper. She is Italian and occasionally, when she is excited, it is difficult to get a clear picture of what she is saying.

"A job!!! It ees a job for Kerena!!!" she cried, waving her newspaper in the air. "There is play in London. They want deaf actresses! Kerena is good actress; she's pretty, so she will get a part."

It sounded very simple put like that. From the newspaper, mum and I discovered that the original American cast of the West End play *Children of a Lesser God* were leaving, and the management was auditioning deaf British actors and actresses to take their place in the play which was about a deaf girl who falls in love with her hearing teacher. With my experience of acting at school, Rosalie and mum were convinced that I'd have a chance of getting a part.

"But I don't have an Equity card!" I wailed.

"Who cares about that?" said mum. Rosalie echoed her.

"Nothing ventured, nothing gained," said dad when he came home.

So next day I turned up at the Albery Theatre, clutching the well-waved-around newspaper. I was not alone, and most of the people clustering around the stage-door had Equity cards. Those of us without couldn't even audition. To soften our disappointment the company invited us all to an open day and a free performance of the play two weeks later.

On the open day there was a signed and spoken tour of the theatre and all the staff told us about their jobs, even the doorman, who told us how he used to carry messages for Katharine Hepburn and Spencer Tracy, when they were acting in the West End. We met the cast, including Elizabeth Quinn, the deaf American actress who had won an award for her portrayal of Sarah in the play, and Sarah Scott, comedian Terry Scott's daughter, who was also hearing-impaired. The performance was brilliant and heart-rending, and it was signed. This was so well done that I began to see signing in a new light and resolved to learn how to do it as soon as I could. Being brought up in a hearing world, sign language was something I'd missed out on and not felt I needed. For the same reason it was a curiously moving day for me because for the first time I met deaf people of my own age. A few of them, like me, had attended an ordinary school, but most had gone to schools for the deaf. It was wonderful to be able to talk about our mutual communication problems with people who really understood. This was a level of support I had done without by going to a hearing school, and by living solely in the hearing world.

The hearing-impaired world is divided into many separate groups which tend to campaign separately, and this is a shame. We all have the same basic problem and we should be working together. But you can see how these separate factions come about, because we have differing requirements. I grumble at a theatre which boasts of having introduced a loop system, because that benefits the hard-of-hearing but is no use to me. I'd rather a sign-language interpreter. But if the loop is a step on the way to signing, I should welcome it as such.

One thing I do accept is that battling in the hearing world isn't suitable or desirable for every deaf person, and there is no stigma attached to conversing in sign language and not speaking. If I had a deaf child who did not want to become part of a hearing world and was content to realise their career ambition in a manual job, who would I be to say that they ought to do any differently?

That open day at the theatre gave me my first proper contact with deaf people, but indirectly, it led to a job under the Manpower Services Commission scheme in Reading as a field-worker in a survey about the problems of the various hearing-impaired communities: the deaf, the deafened and the hard-of-hearing.

I was to meet many of the friends I made at the Albery Theatre again, when I returned from Reading to London and was working in the Subtitling Unit. They were by now members of a deaf drama group called the 66 Club. After a successful spoken, signed and danced production of *The Boyfriend*, they decided to be more ambitious and try *West Side Story*. The music was more complex, and the West-Side dialect very difficult to put into sign language, but they were undaunted. I got roped in to play Rosalia, the homesick Puerto-Rican girl. Acting a part, dancing and speaking and signing was a tremendous strain; it was like doing ten things at once. Every dance routine had to be carefully timed, and counted – if one person went wrong, everyone went out! Luckily we had professional choreographers to help us. We also had professional singers to dub for us. But this was just as difficult as singing, because the singing and the signs had to be in perfect time, and you couldn't watch the singer. You had to count in your head and watch the hearing person in the orchestra keeping the official count and cueing everyone.

Doing this musical showed me just how relevant music is to the deaf, who can feel it and maybe even hear a few frequencies, and it gave me the incentive to have those lessons with my friend James which gave me a foundation for subtitling, singing and the confidence for coping with the hymns in *Songs of Praise*.

My earlier experience of the dole had been brief compared to that of the young Liverpool unemployed I was talking to those days in November. And I had been single, with supportive parents behind me. I didn't have a family of my own to feed and worry about. But even my limited experience of being jobless was a help when talking to youngsters whose families were suffering long-term unemployment or who were struggling to find a job themselves.

Now somehow we had to fill the Cathedral of Christ the King with them without the machinery of the education authority to help get us organised. We decided to record at a weekend and pray that interested teachers and enthusiastic pupils would come in their free time. We rallied the teachers, youth leaders, and clergy, but we could do no more.

On the Saturday, we couldn't believe it! At nine a.m. sharp, the cathedral filled up with youngsters proudly wearing their school uniforms. They got down to work with a singular dedication as we recorded the hymns, unrehearsed for once. We gave them an hour for lunch. "That's the end of that lot," said a sceptical member of the crew. But he was wrong! At two p.m. the children had taken their places to continue. We recorded all the hymns on time and the singing was marvellous! A tribute to Liverpool! As one young interviewee in the programme said to me, "We're young and Liverpudlian and we've lived here all our lives and want to stay here. And if people could believe in Liverpool and in us, we could stay here, and have jobs."

# 10

# Paws on the Redway

Christmas – Skipper's second Christmas with me – was drawing near, so Ruth, Jennifer and I decided to go Christmas shopping in Milton Keynes. I took Skipper with us, but was worrying about leaving him on his own in the car for a long time, as it was rather cold. "But don't you take Skipper shopping with you?" Ruth asked.

I mumbled something about how only Guide Dogs were admitted into shopping complexes.

"Well, I think you should always take Skipper with you, especially at this time of year. He'd tell you if there was a bomb scare or a fire-alarm." This observation made me remember the time I was Christmas shopping in Kensington High Street when there was a bomb alert. Everybody had started to run in all directions and, as I could not hear what was going on, I had absolutely no idea why people were running or from what. If I'd had Skipper, he'd have been able to tell me where the sound was coming from and I could have run in the opposite direction!

Luckily I had Skipper's Hearing-Dog certificate with me in Milton Keynes, so we boldly walked him past the sign which said "No Dogs. Guide Dogs Excepted," and into the shopping complex.

Nobody said anything for quite a while and I started to enjoy shopping, until an assistant in Marks and Spencer came running after me, shouting, "Take that dog out!" I didn't hear her. Ruth did, and explained that I couldn't hear and that Skipper was a Hearing Dog. The assistant seemed satisfied with this explanation, but before I'd finished shopping in Marks three other assistants had asked me to take Skipper out, and I had to produce his certificate. Before long I only had to see an assistant, see her eyes light up as she advanced in our direction to know that this was another dog attack. Worried that they'd make a scene, as nearly happened in C & A, I soon ceased to enjoy what should have been a relaxed afternoon.

I didn't object to being asked why Skipper was there. Hearing Dogs are still a new idea to most people, and being of any breed, they aren't as easy to identify as Guide Dogs. It was the manner in which we were challenged which was upsetting: "Take that dog out!" or "No dogs allowed in this store!"

Many elderly owners of Hearing Dogs feel intimidated by such incidents. Owing to poor speech or a lack of confidence, they are unable to explain why they have a dog with them and, scared by the insensitive attitude of shop assistants, they no longer take their dogs shopping with them. Indeed, if I had not had Ruth and Jennifer with me to make light of the "dog attacks" I don't think I'd have persevered in Milton Keynes.

Skipper, however, was quite enjoying himself. He walked to heel all the time, sat in the queues, and endeared himself to many of the shoppers who recognised him from a scene-stealing photo which accompanied a piece John Craven had written in the *SuperStore Year Book*. All the same, he looked really pleased when I abandoned shopping and took him for a walk.

Skipper and I were staying the weekend with Ruth, and as she has two rather reserved, but self-centred cats, called Rita and Brenda, Skipper was in competition for attention. Rita, Brenda and Skipper spent most of their time casting long penetrating stares at each other. But Rita and Brenda noticed that Skipper got a lot of fuss made of him when he answered the phone, so when the phone rang next, Skipper was stopped in his tracks when there sitting in front of it was Brenda, glaring at him beadily and defying him to come any nearer.

Skipper stopped dead, and quivered. Brenda did not move. What a dilemma for Skipper! But his sense of duty overcame his nervousness of Brenda and he shot round her to the phone. I couldn't but admire his dedication. It reminded me of the day I left him in the office while I went to the restaurant and returned to see him almost sitting on my phone. "Your phone's ringing and Skipper's frantic," someone said as I was about to tell Skipper off for sitting on the desk. But he looked so relieved to see me, as if to say, I thought if I sat on the phone it would keep ringing until you got here.

Despite having to put up with the two cats, Skipper enjoyed staying with Ruth, especially when he got taken for a long walk on Hampstead Heath, which must be his favourite place in London. It made up for Milton Keynes which hadn't left too favourable an impression on either of us. So imagine my feelings when David Kremer announced my next *Songs of Praise* assignment was, of all places, Milton Keynes and it was to be broadcast from the Middleton Hall in the shopping centre. "Well, I'm not going there!" I told him.

"What's wrong with doing a *Songs of Praise* in a shopping centre?" he asked.

I told him what had happened when we had gone Christmas shopping there. David is a champion of the cause of Hearing Dogs. If Skipper is not allowed in a hotel, or if we encounter any problems, it is David who tactfully explains the situation and eventually gets Skipper admitted. The shopping centre was no exception, and the centre manager could not have sounded more helpful when David spoke to him on the phone.

That taught me not to think the worst of people! But I still had doubts about Milton Keynes as a town. "I've been to Milton Keynes quite a few times," I told David, "and I've never seen a church spire. Is it a godless place?"

"Go and find out," was his answer.

I arranged to meet the churches' media officer first. "If there's a media officer, there must be at least one church somewhere," I thought.

Milton Keynes is made for *Songs of Praise* researchers! It's impossible to get lost there. All the estates are on an American grid system and everywhere is so well signposted – and there's no speed limit or traffic lights, except in the older parts and in the centre of town. Pedestrians walk down the redways: footpaths well away from the roads. If I was a child, I could ride a bicycle here, I thought, remembering the restrictions my parents had put on my cycle riding as a child. "You can't ride on the roads, because of the cars. You won't hear them," was their constant warning. When I got a bicycle at university, my dad bought me a wing mirror for it, so that I could see cars behind me. Redways were ideal for children and deaf cyclists.

They were also made for disabled people in wheelchairs. "I can go anywhere, as long as my batteries don't run out!" disabled people told me. "I can get to any level in the shopping centre. They even have wheelchairs you can borrow if you've come in a long way by car."

I arrived early for my meeting with the churches' media officer because parking was no problem. There are hundreds of parking spaces, including disabled-parking areas, all around the shopping centre. I took Skipper for a quick walk down a nearby redway, and then put on the Authorised Dog badge thoughtfully sent us by the centre manager, and walked him into the complex.

I learnt a number of things that afternoon, and one was not to make premature judgments about a place again. The churches' media officer, Barry Amiss, explained the lack of church spires very simply. The emphasis in Milton Keynes is on ecumenical community churches which meet in local halls and on smaller house churches, meeting in people's homes. But in a few years' time there will be a spire in the centre of Milton Keynes, when the Ecumenical Church of Christ the Cornerstone is finally built on the site reserved for it and the existing Church of Christ the Cornerstone can move out of the library, where it is cramped with its constantly expanding congregation.

As I went around meeting more people I also learnt how the church filled some social gaps in a new city lacking the legacies and charities established in older communities over the centuries. The churches were to the fore in things like pensioners' clubs and beds for the homeless and there was a great recycling-absolutely-everything scheme called CROP which gave its profits to local charities. Milton Keynes was full of surprises.

One of them was saved for Skipper. Usually I have to hunt for a place to walk him, but with all these redways and parks everywhere, Skipper was walked off his paws! We walked down one redway, only to find a field of cows. Skipper was terrified of them! What odd cows, I thought, thinking how stiff they looked. They didn't move an inch as we drew closer. Then I remembered and laughed! "They're concrete," I told Skipper. He warily circled the cows, and came no nearer. Concrete or not, he was taking no chances!

Despite his encounter with the concrete cows, Skipper missed the redway walking when we returned to London. "Don't worry," I assured him, "we'll go shopping there more often!" I carefully put Skipper's badge away wondering what problems we were going to encounter and overcome next in our travels with *Songs of Praise*.

# 11

# Friends in Need

British Rail may let Skipper travel free, but it doesn't always make life easy for deaf travellers. I've already mentioned the lip-reading problem with ticket office grilles, but small railway stations could display their names more frequently and prominently down the platforms, and when you have to change trains in a hurry visual information about connections would be useful, not just to the deaf but to all those who find difficulty understanding the station tannoy.

Then there was the time I was travelling overnight to Edinburgh and the attendant refused to let Skipper share the sleeping compartment with me, despite my explanations of why I needed him, and showing his Hearing-Dog certificate and his letter from the British Rail officer for the disabled. There was a real battle as I tried to save Skipper from the guard's van. The station manager and the sleeping-car attendant were adamant that dogs went in the guard's van, not in the sleeping compartment. Luckily, a BBC film crew Skipper and I had worked with were by pure chance boarding the same train, overheard the row, and came to our rescue. The presence of a muscular film crew threatening to film the proceedings provoked a rapid change of heart in the British Rail officials and Skipper and I were allowed to share our sleeper.

Afterwards I wrote to BR to complain and got a most understanding apology which resulted in Skipper and me starring in a BR training video to help staff appreciate the problems of the disabled. This was good news for

Hearing Dogs and, as the officer for the disabled said, "At least *you'll* be recognised in future!" The filming at Euston took forever because the actor playing the part of a BR station supervisor kept being accosted by the travelling public wanting to know where the Ladies was or platform 13 or the time of the next train to Liverpool. But it was all great fun and certainly showed me BR at its caring best.

For me, however, the big test comes when what BR like to call "unforeseen circumstances" intervene, like when the direction board at Victoria had broken down when I was trying to go to Petersfield for *Songs of Praise*. I asked everybody in sight if I was getting on the right train and then asked the ticket inspector if I was in the right half. I wasn't. Skipper and I collected up our luggage and tottered forward and asked him again to make sure.

A nice young man with a packet of crisps got on and Skipper soon made overtures. Before long I was telling him all about Hearing Dogs and what I did and where I was going.

"But this half of the train isn't going to Petersfield," he said. At that I panicked. There was supposed to be a car meeting the train for me and now I'd have to try and phone BBC Transport from somewhere without any special phone equipment.

"Don't worry," Skipper's new friend said, reassuringly knowledgeable. "Get off at the next stop and in about fifteen minutes there's a train that will take you back to Petersfield. I'll make sure you get to the right platform, and don't worry about the car. I'll phone your BBC transport people for you from the station." My worries began to dissolve, and we got off at the next station. It was only then that I remembered my manners and asked if he had been getting off anyway. "No," he replied honestly. "But don't worry, I'm out of work so I'm in no hurry and only too happy to help. Honest. This is making my day interesting." I still felt very guilty. True to his word, the kind man rang Transport and saw me on the right train. I never knew his name and I'm

107

sure I was in too much of a state at the time to think straight and thank him properly.

When I eventually arrived in Petersfield, the hired car was waiting and my worries were almost over. Almost, because I had not yet been able to book a hotel. The few I had contacted had either been shut for the winter or had refused to take Skipper. I now had an hour and a half to find one. I can't remember how many bed and breakfasts I called on, and I was getting further and further out of town. I was having visions of sleeping in the car, when I eventually saw a pub called the Rakeland Arms, which did B & B. "Do you take dogs?" I asked hopefully as a soppy-looking Labrador peered out from behind the bar. "Yes, of course, no problem," replied the cheerful lady. I was so relieved!

Hotels have always been a problem, but when they are willing to have Skipper, they really do do their best to make him happy. I'll never forget the York and Faulkner in Sidmouth, where they managed to squeeze me in to a small room without a bathroom and went on to explain apologetically that there was a two-pound charge for dogs. "But that includes his evening meal which is bits of whatever is on the menu, and will he require breakfast?" I think the York is now Skipper's favourite hotel, because every morning he would wake up wagging his tail waiting for me to take his bowl to the kitchens, while he sat outside waiting for whatever gastronomic delights that were going to be in his bowl – chicken, beef, sausage, the list was endless!

So many things happen to Skipper and me when we are out researching and I have learnt that, while you may get a misunderstanding here or there, the majority of complete strangers are only too happy to make allowances and be helpful if only I will let them. Petersfield was no exception. The first potential disaster was saved by the young man with the crisps, and the people I had appointments to meet did everything to ensure I ate a succession of teas and suppers, organised my phone calls for me, and one even offered me her own bed. Nobody said, "She's deaf, she shouldn't be doing a job which requires so much use of the phone." Indeed, everywhere I go there is always someone who says they get so much pleasure making calls for me – Christine in Haddington, Anne in Dumfries, Dilys in Aberystwyth, and in Petersfield Canon Cyril Taylor, composer of the famous hymn tune "Abbot's Leigh" which usually accompanies "Glorious things of thee are spoken". The list is endless. Not only do these people go out of their way to help, but their interest is sparked, and I know the special relationship I am able to strike up with them helps me achieve a greater depth to my research. If I was not deaf and did not have Skipper I would not find out half the things or meet half the people I do.

Lip-reading takes a great deal of concentration. Towards the end of the day you become tired and less able to understand what is being said. Once when I had had a long day in the office and was looking forward to a quiet evening at home with just Skipper for company. An evening with Skipper is very relaxing. When you talk to him he moves his head from side to side as if he understands everything you say and replies with little doggy gestures that you don't have to lip-read. We were just about to leave the office, when I remembered it was somebody's leaving party that evening and I couldn't not go to it. It was the last thing that I felt like! I took Skipper home, fed him, and made my way to the wine bar alone.

Wine bars are not the ideal places for deaf people. Background noise and loud music makes partially hearing people unable to hear a conversation. That does not bother me – I manage better than most at a noisy party – but what does make things difficult in a wine bar is the poor light, especially after a tiring day. As usual, a place had been saved for me in the middle of the table where I could see everybody. During the meal I made a few efforts to join in the conversation, but gradually pretended that my meal was more absorbing. I didn't feel a part of the occasion. I felt like someone must feel when all the other people are speaking a different language, and I became more aware of the division between the deaf and hearing worlds. I have always seen myself as a person who happens to be deaf, not as a deaf person. But at that moment I felt like a deaf person who would have rather talked in sign language. But this reminded me that sometimes when I have gone out with a group of deaf friends talking in sign language, I have felt the same kind of isolation. Sign language is very much a second language for me and at times I can get quite lost in a signed conversation. There are two worlds, I thought, and I don't belong in either. I go between the two, not quite fitting in. I remembered a party I once had when my deaf friends stood at one end of the room and signed and my hearing friends chatted normally at the other end and I ran between the two trying to integrate them.

Occasionally I feel deaf and this was one of the times. Unable to follow the conversation, I felt lonely and cut off. It took me until the next morning to realise that I was far from being lonely and cut off with friends who really did care and take the trouble to communicate with me. But, in the next few weeks, I learned what real loneliness was.

It was Help the Aged's Silver Jubilee and we were doing a *Songs of Praise* to mark that occasion. Help the Aged was founded as a charity to help elderly victims of overseas disasters. It is always the children who win people's hearts and are at the front of the queue for relief supplies. The elderly, if they are at all able to reach the refugee camps, are too weak to even join a food queue. "I asked if there were any elderly people in the camp," one Help-the-Aged worker told me, "and I was told there weren't. I looked in the tents and found starving old people crouching at the back."

Researching our programme, I realised exactly why the charity has also felt the need to turn its attentions nearer home. Loneliness is perhaps the most shocking problem of old age. I visited one lady who had sat for a week in darkness because a light bulb had failed and she could not change it. Another had been unable to pull herself out of a bath and had lain there for a weekend. Another had become a prisoner in her own

110

flat at the top of a tower block for six weeks when the lift was vandalised. One of the worst cases I saw was a lady who had nobody and just stared at four walls. When she went out to get her pension a gang of youths followed her back and she was mugged and raped.

I realised too that many an elderly, house-bound person in need of friendship was too proud to ask for it. "The last person I saw was the postman, when he delivered a parcel to me for next-door," one lady wrote to Help the Aged.

What, I asked myself severely, was I doing being sorry for myself and feeling deaf and lonely?

I always thought that I would have problems with film crews – I don't know why, but I did. I was proved very wrong . . . The first time I took Skipper filming the camera crew gave him a look as if to say, if you keep running into shot, you're in for it. Skipper was good that first morning, sitting patiently behind the camera. His only misdemeanour was scratching by the sound man's microphone, and drowning Roger Royle's link about Aberystwyth. But he never did it again and observes the rule of absolute silence during filming, like the professional he is. Skipper loves filming! The film crews enjoy playing with him. Sometimes they are even grateful to him! Once we went to film holiday-makers supposedly having a good time on the beach of a popular holiday resort. As there was nobody doing this because of the poor weather and we couldn't change the filming time, we were desperate. Then, the camera man spotted Skipper happily digging a stone into the sand and turned and filmed him – the happy "holiday-maker"!

Another time when we were filming an open-air *Songs of Praise* in the grounds of a ruined castle, there were so many people milling round, the camera men and stage managers kept losing the people they were meant to film singing the hymns they had chosen. As Skipper had met them all whilst researching, he was soon roped in to help. "Find Mark!" "Find Carol!" "Find Lisa," the camera man or stage manager would say and Skipper would trot into the thick of the congregation, hunting the person in question.

Roger Royle, one of our presenters, is a great fan of Skipper – and somebody who has always encouraged and supported me. In my early days in *Songs of Praise*, he was always full of helpful advice. He is always cheerful and genuinely interested in the people he interviews, and good at putting them at ease. He is also very sensitive to other people's problems. "I don't know a great deal about deafness," he informed me on our first meeting, "but I suppose communication must take a great deal of concentration and you must get tired easily. If that happens, don't be polite! Don't feel that you have to struggle on to understand me – give in."

For the Christmas *Songs of Praise* I had the idea of dressing Roger up as Father Christmas in the toy department of a big store and then he went to give out presents in the children's ward of a hospital. Another time I arranged for him to travel from London to Aberystwyth in a hurry by helicopter, not realising how much he hated flying. He now tends to greet me with a wary, "And what has your research landed me in for this time?" And I have yet to answer to Cliff Michelmore for obliging him to interview a thatcher while clinging tenaciously to the top of a ladder.

When I had been at *Songs of Praise* for about three months I began to work out where my problems lay. Partly, they were of my own making. I suppose I had been trying so hard to make people forget I was deaf that sometimes they really did and would talk to me when my back was turned or say without thinking things like, "Take the tape and listen to it on my Walkman."

My trouble has always been that I'm very bad about asking for help and I'd have saved myself a lot of trouble and frustration if I'd been more honest about my difficulties to start off with. But I didn't want them to think I couldn't cope and I desperately wanted to be asked to stay on for another six months.

Every two weeks there was a *Songs of Praise* meeting to discuss the programmes which had been broadcast.

Meetings are one of the situations I have the greatest difficulty with. People speak quickly, and subjects and speakers change rapidly. Once I've found the next speaker, by looking, they've usually almost finished speaking and the subject has changed, so I've got to find out what the new subject is. To make matters worse, comments are usually addressed to the chair, so either you sit by the person chairing the meeting, and catch the comments addressed to them, but not what they say, or you sit opposite them and follow what they say but miss out on the comments.

I resolved not to worry about actually following in the meetings, but to ask what had been said afterwards. This would bring a puzzled reaction. "But you were in the meeting, weren't you?" Of course I was, even if I couldn't follow! As they'd never encountered me in a situation where I couldn't cope, their answer was understandable.

The only time I asked for help was with taking names and addresses and dates on the phone. Everyone is superb about doing that. I don't even have to ask. When I make a call, someone is always at hand to mouth what is being said on the phone if I need help. The one thing I hate is answerphones because I never know when to begin talking, but I know most of my hearing friends dislike chatting to answerphones too. You listen to yourself sounding silly.

My main problem as far as phones were concerned was that I was sharing a line with several other people and when they were busy and not thinking, they'd answer the phone before Skipper had a chance to tell me. This began to put his nose out of joint, and confused him. Am I responsible for this phone or not? he must have been wondering, so he began not always to answer the phone, which was worrying for me. Another problem with sharing a line was that I never knew if someone was already using it, so I'd frequently cut them off. What finally made me decide that I had to have a phone of my own was when one of our young interviewees rang me from a call box and I promised to call back.

Before I could do so, someone else was using the line, and as that was the only one with my special phone, I was stuck. I felt so sorry for the poor person in the call box, getting colder and colder and wondering why I didn't call back and I really began to feel disabled.

It was a combination of all these things that finally made me decide to say something to Stephen Whittle, I had to screw myself up to do it, remembering the school teacher I'd asked not to face the blackboard when talking to us. "Well, if you can't cope in a normal school, you had better go to a school for the deaf," had been her response. So I waited a long time before telling Stephen about the problems I was having in the office, worrying unnecessarily about them.

Once I'd plucked up the courage to speak, things were soon put right. Someone agreed to take notes for me at meetings. Skipper and I had a telephone line to ourselves, and when people heard an answerphone on my amplified telephone, they'd tell me when the tone came and what the message said. Really, the problems I was having were not caused by insensitivity but forgetfulness. As one colleague said, "I forget that you're deaf until I ask you something when your back is turned, or see Skipper rushing to answer the phone."

"I never know what to do at times," Jan, one of our production assistants, told me. "I sometimes see you struggling to do something and want to help, but then I think that if I offer to help you'll feel patronised. I just wish you would sometimes swallow your pride and ask for help." Jan was right, I am too ready to think that asking for help is to admit failure, yet I am always very happy to help a person in a wheel-chair out of difficulties or help a blind person over the road, and would never attribute having to help them to failure on their part. One of the problems when you're deaf is that people can't see that you are having problems, unless the frustration and lack of comprehension is very obvious, so you do have to ask for help or explain and, to be honest, I do at times find this humiliating.

"You will always have problems at work," Sheila, one

of the supervisors on the MSC project I worked on in Reading, warned me. "But you will always be able to overcome them by yourself or with the help of others." And I certainly got a lot of help in Reading before I joined the BBC. Sheila and her colleague, Paul, would spend hours helping me to use an amplified phone in the office. They made sure that I had the most powerful hearing-aids going and made me aware of all the special equipment available to help deaf people.

They also taught me that asking for help can make other people's jobs more rewarding and interesting. One day I gave up typing, frustrated. "What's wrong?" asked Peter, a young worker on the MSC scheme with cerebral palsy.

"I can't hear the bell go when I get to the end of the line and I'm ending up with half-typed words and a bottle of Tipp-Ex all over this page," I explained.

Peter, who loved inventing things, looked thoughtful. The next week he came into work with a small present for me. I opened it and inside was a funny-looking device with a light on it. "You fix it to the typewriter like this," he explained and when the carriage-return hits the bell the light will come on. So, no more typing mistakes!" The device worked well and Peter tried to have it patented, but did not have the money to do so, which is sad because it was invaluable for me and could have helped so many other deaf typists.

Remembering the kind people in Reading made me wonder why I was being so silly about seeking help from the equally understanding people in *Songs of Praise*. "I don't know why you don't have more confidence in yourself," Stephen told me. "You're doing fine and we're going to give you another six months here. Let that give you confidence and always tell me if something is not right."

Getting a six-month extension certainly built up my confidence. I started to interrupt in meetings and own up to not following. I asked for help and this meant people knew when to come to my aid without being asked and without feeling that they were patronising me. And I was happier than I had ever been, knowing that I was succeeding in a different part of the BBC which involved working with the public. I knew that I still had a long way to go, but I was determined to make a success of working in production. I had enjoyed subtitling, but the long, lonely hours at a TV monitor, working on a programme that had already been made, was not as challenging as participating in the making of one. I loved meeting people in connection with *Songs of Praise*; they always have an effect on me. I can be feeling really depressed about something and meet a cheerful person, who has nothing to be cheerful about, and their happiness washes onto me and makes me realise that my problems are very minor. It also gives me the confidence that, especially on a one-to-one basis, I can hold a conversation with anyone and am a normal person who happens to be deaf, not just a deaf person.

# 12

## Riot Estate to Stately Homes

Originally, Hearing Dogs for the Deaf had been under the auspices of the RNID. But now it was a separate charity in its own right! To celebrate the occasion, a reception was held in London, to which Skipper and I were invited. We were both determined to go, especially when Gillian rang to say Stella was going to be awarded a badge as a thank-you for her fund-raising efforts. "But don't tell her, because she and Mike are coming anyway and it will be a surprise for her."

As Skipper was the wagging, licking, breathing result of Stella's work, I gave him a good brush to make sure he did her credit. He looked so smooth and sleek when I'd finished – but not for long! Quite disgusted with his new image, he zealously shook himself. Not content with that, he rolled on the floor until his fur really did stand up on end. "Oh Skipper!" I wailed. "Look at you!" He just peered up as if to say, if you can go about with a punk haircut, why can't I? I had a feeling he was in a cheeky mood.

When we arrived at the reception and Skipper saw people he knew and, most important, saw food, his ears pricked up and he trotted off to say hello to his friends. So much for my escort! At least he had the courtesy to talk to both his human and canine friends.

I found myself being introduced to a number of potential fund-raisers, who were all interested in knowing how Skipper had changed my life. I was in the middle of explaining, when out of the corner of my eye I saw

Skipper bound across the room. Stella and her husband, Mike, had arrived.

When the speeches started, I made sure that Skipper and I were standing where we could see Stella, right in the front. Skipper was confused. He had been sure that this was a party, not a meeting, and speeches just did not happen at parties. With all his friends around, especially Gillian's dog, Gemma, he had no wish whatsoever to sit still. It was all I could do to persuade him to sit like a wobbly jelly, which was a far cry from his normal statue-still meeting-behaviour at work.

Suddenly, Skipper got up, went to the front where all could see him and rolled onto his back, sticking his legs in the air. This untypical behaviour was very embarrassing, especially as everyone was laughing at the ridiculous creature, and worse still, looking in its owner's direction. Later Gillian explained that in his speech the president of the RNID, Lord Chalfont, had said how clever and well trained Hearing Dogs were, and indicated Skipper and Gemma. Skipper must have heard the word dog and decided to go and take a bow.

Not only did Skipper understand the speech, he also seemed to be able to lip-read. When he sneaked over to play with Gemma during another speech, and Gillian crossly mouthed, "Go and sit next to Kerena!" he slunk back to me.

Thankfully, Skipper's manners began to improve and when the flabbergasted Stella went up to accept her award, he did not, as I had feared, try and sneak in another bow for himself. He just sat and smiled his doggy smile. Skipper and I were so pleased for her because it is one thing for an organisation to raise a lot of money, but for an individual like Stella to do so demands a singular dedication.

One of the things that people always ask me on occasions like this is, "Does Skipper do things that he is not trained to do?" He does so often that I tend to forget specific incidents. When someone puts newspapers through the door, if someone falls over the milk bottles, if a car-alarm goes off in the street, Skipper uses

his initiative and comes and takes me to the source of
the new sound. Some dogs just do what they're trained
to do, but others will use their initiative, especially if the
owner has complete trust and always leaves things to
the dog, ignoring people who try to tell the owner about
the sound the dog will respond to. This helps the dog
to recognise that its owner depends on it and it often
tries to please the owner by responding to new sounds.
I depend utterly on Skipper and make a big fuss of him
when he does something, so he really seems to enjoy
using his initiative.

When we got home after the reception, I was just
about to start the cooking when I felt a little paw urgently
tap my leg. "What is it?" I asked. Skipper replied by
trotting off into the lounge, past the phone – so it wasn't
the phone – and stopped by the coat hanger. My coat
had fallen off the hanger. As I picked the coat up and
put it back, Skipper smiled happily. Obviously this was
an important sound because I had done something about
it. I wondered if he was storing it away in his doggy
brain. He was even more pleased when I gave him a
lump of his favourite cheese as a well-earned reward
and played with him.

Soon after the reception Gillian invited Skipper and
me to visit the new enlarged premises Hearing Dogs for
the Deaf had moved into at Lewknor, not far from their
first home at Chinnor. They now had a bungalow in a
delightful apple orchard, a stable block awaiting conver-
sion when they could raise more funds, kennels in
need of repair and expansion and a caravan donated by
Andrex to take to dog shows and country fairs to tell
people about what they did. Tony and Gillian were
clearly on the brink of an ambitious programme of expansion that would need a lot of funds. They had come
a long way in four years.

"Did I ever tell you," Gillian said, "that before we had
Chinnor we used to have to train the first dogs in my
landlady's dining-room?'

"What happened when you wanted to give a dinner
party?"

"We didn't have any!"

Many more dogs have been placed with deaf recipients since Skipper, the thirteenth dog, came to open up my world. It was so exciting to stand in the kennels and see what the future could hold for Hearing Dogs. I felt sure that the day would come when the orange-coloured leads and collars would be as recognisable as the Guide Dogs' harness and Hearing Dogs for the Deaf would be as familiar as Guide Dogs for the Blind.

All Saints' Church, Edmonton was celebrating its 850th year and had invited us to do a *Songs of Praise* there to mark this occasion. On the north side of the North Circular, surrounded by furniture warehouses and busy roads, the traditional church and graveyard of All Saints is dwarfed by tower blocks. We decided not only to invite the Edmonton churches but also those from Edmonton's neighbours: the middle-class Enfield, as well as Tottenham, where we could see how the residents of the Broadwater Farm estate were getting on a few months after the notorious riots. It was definitely an interesting assignment and I was pleased that I was to research it.

"Don't go walking around the Broadwater Farm estate on your own," Simon, the producer, warned. "I'll be back from holiday in a few weeks' time and I'll go round it with you."

At first I thought that this was a good idea, but I soon got impatient to research that particular area. "If I'm too scared to go there, I shouldn't be doing the job," I told myself sternly and decided to spend an afternoon on the estate getting the feeling of the place.

We drove down Mount Pleasant Road, where some of the rioting had taken place and a few burnt-down houses near the Methodist church marked one of the entrances to the Broadwater Farm. "Here we go," I told Skipper as we drove on to the estate and parked the car.

I was getting Skipper's lead out of the car boot, when I felt someone standing behind me. I turned around and saw a policeman. "What are those for?" he asked, pointing to the box of empty bottles I carry around in my car in the hope that I will find a bottle bank to put them in. To him empties meant petrol bombs. I explained, and told him what I was doing on the estate.

The Broadwater Farm estate was not what I expected it to be. Despite the grey blocks of flats, it was surrounded by a park and a children's playground. Bunches of fresh flowers marked the spot where PC Blakelock fell. Under the blocks of flats were parking spaces, which could be spooky on a dark night. As Skipper and I wandered about, the policemen walking around in pairs were very obvious, but they would pause to chat with the residents every now and then, and there certainly was not the oppressive atmosphere I had expected to find, even if the burnt-out shops were a reminder of what had happened a few months previously.

Having got the feeling of the place, I went back to the office to think about the kind of people I would start looking for. I also went through the newspaper and TV reports of the riots, hoping to find some inspiration there. There was the elderly lady, who did not know the riots were going on because she was watching *Songs of Praise*. I resolved to find her and also wanted to find a West-Indian family and a policeman. The local Methodist minister knew the *Songs of Praise* lady and offered to take me to meet some other interesting people.

His church was right outside the estate and the riots had taken place during the Sunday evening service. Quite a number of families had taken refuge in the church that night. One of these that I was introduced to was the West-Indian family who lived on top of the Asian supermarket that was burnt down. Everyone was at church or at work except the father, who was also watching *Songs of Praise* at the time of the riot. "I heard nothing," he told me, "until *Songs of Praise* had finished. I'd been recording it for the family on the video. There was a knock at the door and a neighbour said, 'Get out, the supermarket's on fire underneath you.'" When the family returned the next day, the thick concrete floor had prevented the fire from spreading, but many things in the flat, except some videos of *Songs of Praise*, which

121

they showed me, had melted with the intense heat. "But we wouldn't live anywhere else," the family assured me. "There's a lovely atmosphere here and now the riots are over it's great. It wasn't the residents who started it; it was outsiders. We'd see people in the corridors, lurking around. Now they aren't here any more."

Other residents confirmed the theory that the rioters were outsiders. They had noticed a number of people coming into the estate on that fateful day and had seen them escape through the estate park and over a wire fence at the back once the trouble had started. Most residents agreed that the police presence was keeping these people out of the estate now.

Every resident I spoke to I asked the same question. "Do you know of a policeman that I could talk to?" They all told me about the same man, but nobody seemed to know his name. He was local. He had been badly injured, trying to save PC Blakelock. He was a Christian and had done a lot towards building better relations between the police and the community by giving talks in church halls. When I finally did track him down I was not disappointed. "I was so close to being killed that night," he told us, "and only God's grace and the bravery of my colleagues saved me." He was sure God had saved his life for a reason. At the time that we spoke to him, his scars were healing and he was gradually coming to terms with his internal injuries. He had seen PC Blakelock viciously knifed to death, had bricks hurled at him and himself fallen under a knife attack. During that time his thoughts were of his family and what would happen to them. Now his thoughts were of the community and his hopes that society would work towards getting rid of the prejudices and ignorance that cause people to go out and maim each other.

The burnt-out Asian supermarket was a tragic reminder of who bore the brunt of the riots. For many reasons, the Asians are the odd ones out in race relations. Walking around the Broadwater it was painfully easy to tell an Asian flat by the graffiti scrawled all over the doors. It saddened me that I spent some time trying to find a Christian Asian family to choose a hymn, and that they were either non-existent or still hiding behind closed doors and burglar-alarms.

Most residents had chains and alarms which frequently went off accidentally. Poor Skipper would run round and round me, thinking that a fire-alarm had gone off. "Is there a fire?" I asked a policeman when he first did this.

"It's only a burglar-alarm," he explained as I carried the confused dog off the estate.

You meet everybody working on *Songs of Praise* and go everywhere and I suppose it's not everybody who has to visit a family on the Broadwater Farm and then rush off to see the Earl of Lauderdale in the House of Lords. But, that is all part of a day's work, and really goes to show that we work with everybody. I had to visit the Earl because we were doing a programme from Haddington, just east of Edinburgh. The Earl had revived an ancient pilgrimage from the village of Whitekirk to the shrine of Our Lady and the Kilted Magi in the Lauderdale aisle in St Mary's church, Haddington. Apart from being one of the few churches in the Church of Scotland to have a pilgrimage attached to it, St Mary's was interesting for a number of other reasons. Destroyed by warring Scots and English armies during the sixteenth century, it was restored in 1971, for "the glory of God and the solace of the whole community, that all may be one". True to that promise, there are Catholic and Episcopal chapels in St Mary's under the roof of the Church of Scotland.

Soon after our visit to the Earl of Lauderdale, Skipper and I left Tottenham and Edmonton to research rural Haddington. It was snowing heavily when we left London and I decided to take my ski-ing clothes in case it got worse. We picked up the hire car at Waverley station and drove slowly through the snow-covered roads to Haddington on the edge of the Lammermuir Hills. I began to wonder if I would ever get to Haddington, let alone research it, and when we did we were snowed in.

Christine, the administrator of St Mary's, was relieved to see us. "You must be frozen!" she exclaimed as a snow-covered Skipper and I made puddles all over her office. "I thought you'd never get here. You must have a coffee." Skipper flopped down beside the fire, whilst I warmed my hands on my mug and Christine rang up members of the local congregations for us. "How are you going to get out to visit them?" she asked.

"I'll drive where I can and walk the rest of the way," I replied, realising that I had to see people in Dunbar and North Berwick, both of which were fifteen miles away from Haddington.

Christine gave me a surprised look and continued to make my calls. "She says she'll walk," I saw her explain to one snowed-in person. "Yes, I would have food and coffee for her – and a fire for Skipper."

Christine thought we were both mad as we set off with the Ordnance Survey map, me in moon-boots and ski-suit and Skipper happily chasing the snowballs. When the snow got deeper, he bounced along like a rabbit.

We were to visit Norah who had built an observatory at her farmhouse and rejoiced that modern science was at last finding a way to connect the wonders of astronomy to the concept of God. And we went on to see a retired tweedmaker who wove woollen cloth, which he sold to Liberty's in London, made in the breathtaking colour schemes of the sky and the Lammermuir Hills around him. Next day we visited the Cistercian abbey of Nunraw. The old abbey was now a guest house for people in need of succour and renewal, like alcoholics or drug addicts who wanted space to sort themselves out in peace. But the monks had recently built a new abbey with a marvellous view of Haddington. "We call it the bargain abbey," the abbot told me, "because all our materials are secondhand."

A former Franciscan priory in Haddington was known as the Lamp of the Lothians, because of the example it set and the work that it did in the community. The late Duke and present Dowager Duchess of Hamilton had established a trust in the same name to restore old buildings in the town and turn them into community centres.

The Duchess was very taken with Skipper, and wanted to know all about Hearing Dogs. "You must be exhausted having to lip-read all the time," she remarked. "I know a bit about deafness because Evelyn Glennie, the young deaf percussion player, came and played in a fund-raising concert for the Lamp, and I found her fascinating." I had heard a great deal about Evelyn who, like myself, had gone to a normal school. Despite being deaf she had pursued her love of music and gained a place at the Royal Academy of Music. A skilled percussion player, she aims to establish percussion as a solo instrument in its own right.

Christine at St Mary's had told the Duchess all about my walking through the snow to the outlying farms. "You must come back to Lennoxlove and relax," said the Duchess. "I've got acres of land for Skipper to roam in and you won't feel that you have to make conversation with me. Just have a good rest before you go back to London tonight." Skipper grinned his appreciation. It was not every dog that got invited to roam a stately home, and he knew it.

We were both sad to leave Haddington. The people had accepted us and been an inspiration to us. As we drove back to Edinburgh and our night train, St Mary's church was illuminated against the night sky and the ghostly backdrop of the snow-covered Lammermuir Hills – a true Lamp of the Lothians.

I love the country, but I am very much a city person, who feels more at home amongst tower blocks and cramped terrace houses. Inspiring as Haddington had been, the recording of the hymns at Edmonton and Tottenham was a lamp to the world too, but in a very different way. The church was filled with people from all walks of life – middle-class people from Enfield, tower-block dwellers from Edmonton, Broadwater residents from Tottenham. There were Catholics, Methodists, Baptists, Anglicans and Pentecostals among the congregation. Some policemen were there too. Nobody could fail to be moved when the congregation boldly sang the last hymn:

Let there be peace on earth and let it begin with me;
Let there be peace on earth, the peace that was
    meant to be,
With God as our Father, brothers all are we,
Let me walk with my brother in perfect harmony.

# 13

# Superstar of David

One afternoon when Chris, Simon and I were engrossed in trying to write a script, Kathy and Angela from *SuperStore* came into the office, unnoticed by us. It wasn't us they wanted anyway. They were more interested in Skipper who, bored with script writing, was lovingly nosing David Kremer's knee in the hope of receiving a custard cream.

"Can we pick him up?" Angela asked David, and proceeded to do so. "He's a bit on the heavy side," she commented.

"Well, he's just eaten a custard cream," said David, wondering what this was all about.

"But he does look like a little waif," Kathy said, having her go at heaving a puzzled Skipper off the ground. Whatever it was they wanted they were satisfied that Skipper filled the bill.

"Could his owner come and have a word with us when she's not so busy?" they asked, noticing that the script-writing party did not want to be disturbed.

The whole office was dying with curiosity to know what Skipper could be wanted for by weight and as soon as we'd finished the script I made my way to the *SuperStore* office to find out.

There was, of course, a simple explanation! Every year *SuperStore* have a *Superstars* competition. Hundreds of children from all over the country audition for this and eventually about twenty acts are selected to appear on *SuperStore*, when the viewers vote for the one they like best. Those who are selected come to London, where they rehearse and perform their act, just like professional artists. Louise and Dionne Bushnell, two sisters from Scotland, were going to sing a pathetic song called "Me and little Andy" about a little girl and her puppy Andy, who, abandoned and near to death, are befriended by an old lady on a dark night. Skipper was being auditioned for the part of Andy and all that sample lifting had been to see whether a little girl of eight would be able to pick him up. Skipper was to be an actor! I only hoped that his talents were up to scratch.

The following Saturday a taxi arrived to take Skipper and me to the television rehearsal rooms in Acton. I was beginning to enjoy the VIP treatment, even if I was only chaperone to the star. However, my enjoyment was short lived. When we arrived at Acton, I showed the commissionaire my identity card and Skipper's, but he would not let us in. "But he's a Hearing Dog for the Deaf and he's been issued with a staff identity card because he accompanies me to work," I patiently explained.

"No dogs, miss," the commissionaire gruffly replied.

I was astounded. This was back to square one with a vengeance. I tried to stay calm and went through all the old arguments. "If he was a Guide Dog for the Blind would you let him in?"

"No!" was the adamant reply.

"If I was in a wheel-chair, would you let my chair in?" I was trying very hard to control my temper.

"Yes, because the chair is part of the person," he replied cryptically.

Thankfully, someone from *SuperStore* noticed my predicament and called for the foreman and eventually I was let in. But his attitude was very concessionary and there was no apology. Seldom are there times when insensitivity hurts me, but this was one – I felt disabled, humiliated, frustrated, almost a criminal.

Luckily I knew that this episode was very untypical of the BBC. But what if I had been a deaf or blind visitor, what would I have thought then? I resolved to send a memo to the manager of the rehearsal rooms, then put it out of my mind, though I was still shaking with anger, in order to introduce Skipper to Dionne and Louise, his two co-stars.

We tied string to Skipper's collar, and like a professional actor he assumed a stray-like appearance – his tail down and a lost look in his eyes. "Try to remember how you felt when you were lost in Stow-on-the-Wold," I urged. His co-star, Louise, fed him a few custard creams and he began to look lovingly at her. After a few more custard creams he soon picked up what he had to do.

Skipper was brilliant! He allowed Louise to carry him into Dionne's "cottage"; sat before the fire looking pathetic; and even jumped into bed with Louise when he was told to. I was relieved that he was doing so well, and hoped he would keep it up on the night.

Luckily the recording the following evening was on home ground at Television Centre, so there wouldn't be any problems with the commissionaire over Skipper. When we arrived the previous act had still not finished, so we found some vacant chairs in the studio and watched. Skipper soon grew bored and fell asleep until his call.

I could hardly recognise Dionne, transformed into a kindly old lady, and Louise as a scruffy urchin. But Skipper had no difficulty in recognising them and happily trotted off to inspect the set and have a final rehearsal before the recording. During the rehearsal he looked pathetic and jumped onto the bed at the right time and lay with his head on the pillow, balefully staring at the camera, the epitome of a dying dog. I was sure he was on the way to a doggy Oscar!

If Skipper's performance was impressive, the set was even more so. There was a Victorian cottage, filled with furniture and knick-knacks, while outside the house an artificial snow machine provided a formidable blizzard.

"Never perform with children or animals," is a well-known Thespian expression, and Skipper proved that performing with animals can be a hazard. He was gradually becoming rather bored – he was getting things right and being told to do them again and this was NOT on! He was all right during take one, although his impatience was beginning to register when he jumped

Sounds Like Skipper

on the bed and retreated under the blankets instead of
lying with his head on the pillow.

During take two he was even more difficult and in take
three he gritted his paws on the floor and refused to do
anything. "Just like a brilliant actor would do," commented an actor friend of mine, when he heard the story.

However, Dionne and Louise were delighted with
him. They had been unable to find a well-behaved dog
in the heats, and had not expected as much from Skipper
as I had. They were so grateful for Skipper's help that
they promised me a free hairdo at their mother's hair-
dressing salon next time I was north of the border.

Later on in the week, *SuperStore* invited us to their
office to see the video of "Me and Little Andy". They
had used the best of Skipper from takes one and two,
and the result was not as bad as I had feared.

The day that Louise, Dionne and Skipper's heat of the
*SuperStore Superstars'* competition was to be broadcast,
mum and I sat glued to the screen, finger on the record
button of the video. Skipper, for his part, flew out of
the room as soon as he heard the song start! Whether
this was stage fright or dread of having to do it again or
shame at his dreadful performance, we didn't know,
but he was later found hiding under the bedclothes.

If we thought that Skipper's performance was lacking,
few other people did! After the song, Mike Read interviewed Louise and Dionne. "Did you enjoy doing that?"
he asked.

"Oh, yes!" they replied enthusiastically.

"And did that dog behave itself?" asked Mike, knowing full well that Skipper had not.

"Oh, he was very, very good," Dionne and Louise
replied with Thespian loyalty.

"What nice girls!" mum exclaimed, shrieking with
laughter. "They didn't spill the beans, and they were so
good, Skipper should be ashamed of himself!"

Needless to say Louise and Dionne won their heat hands
down and went through to the finals. They were thrilled
and wrote to Skipper, thanking him for his help. "You'd get
away with murder!" I told him when I read him their letter.

130

He looked at me as if to say, I'm sweet, I don't have to act. Skipper's charms and Louise and Dionne's talent did not win them the final, alas. But the girls were just happy to have taken part. Winning was not everything.

If I thought that was the end of Skipper's career as an actor, I was mistaken. Not long after, Angela and Kathy from *SuperStore Superstars* came back to see us. Skipper gave them a look of warm dread, before he remembered his manners and said hello. "I think he remembers us!" they commented.

"What we wondered," they began, avoiding Skipper's penetrating glare, "is if you would lend Skipper to us for *Children in Need*. We plan to re-record all the *Superstars* entrants as part of the appeal with better sets and proper costumes." I knew Skipper would say no, but as *Children in Need* was such a worthy cause I said yes for him and resolved to have a long talk with him later.

Knowing what a moody star she was dealing with, Angie decided against rehearsing him. "We'll only use him in the takes and that way he won't get fed up." I wished I had more faith in Skipper.

When his call came, I had to coax him onto the set with a bowl of cheese and promises of nice walkies when it was over. I was convinced that he would let everybody down. But, like many temperamental stars, he excelled himself, better than he had ever been before! He sat by the bed, his pathetic eyes saying, I'm going to die if you won't let me stay by your fire and sleep in your bed. At the right moment he lay down on the bed beside Louise and slowly closed his eyes just at the time when the little dog dies. Brilliant!!

But, I looked a sight! "Stand near the camera where he can see you," everyone advised, "so that he looks into the camera." But the best position was in firing range of the artificial snow machine! I looked much more frost bitten than the dying child and little Andy.

"Wonderful! Splendid!" said the producer. He was so pleased with the remake that he asked Skipper and me to appear on *Children in Need*. Skipper gave him a look as if to say, I don't have to go all through that again, do I? "All you need to do is talk about what Skipper does for you," the producer explained. "Skipper need not do anything, and hopefully, Louise and Dionne will be at the Glasgow end that night."

"Well, if it will help *Children in Need*, I'll appear in the studio with pleasure," I replied, wondering how Skipper and I would fit in. Hearing Dogs are not placed with children. What I didn't realise when I made this rash promise was that *Children in Need* was not only live, but unrehearsed!

On the night I was TERRIFIED, knowing that all my friends, relatives and their friends were going to watch. "Me and Little Andy" was the last of the *SuperStore* items, and as soon as Skipper heard the music he stood in a small, miserable heap and looked at me as if to say, not that again, please! I replied by dragging the reluctant hound onto the set.

After the video of the song had finished, Sarah Greene interviewed Louise and Dionne in Glasgow. The girls had been doing a massive fund-raising and made a considerable sum for *Children in Need*. Because I had to sit in-between Sarah and Mike Read, where it was difficult to see what they said, I kept a wary eye on a TV monitor underneath the coffee table, so that I would know when they talked to me. I need not have worried, Sarah turned and faced me, giving me a slight tap. "Skipper is a Hearing Dog for the Deaf and he has his own BBC identity card," Sarah explained as she introduced us. Luckily I had brought Skipper's card with me and she was able to show it to the cameras.

"I could get in on that!" Mike quipped as Skipper happily licked his face. Everything was rushing by in a blur, but I remembered explaining what Skipper did as a Hearing Dog in the BBC.

"How did he take to stardom?" Sarah asked.

"He wasn't a natural actor," I apologised. "If it had not been for Louise and Dionne's patience, I don't think we would ever have made 'Me and Little Andy'." I paid some more tributes to the girls who had had to put up with their temperamental co-star, while Skipper replied by going to sleep on Mike's knee.

"Does he like the song?" Sarah asked.

"Oh, he hates it," I replied truthfully. "Whenever he hears it he goes and hides!" I just hoped that the girls would realise that Skipper had bad taste in music.

Sarah rounded off by explaining that some of the money raised by *Children in Need* would help deaf children, then Sue Cook and Terry Wogan took over. To Skipper's relief "Me and Little Andy" was well and truly over, and so was my ordeal of appearing unrehearsed on a live TV show.

On the domestic front Skipper and I were going through a certain amount of upheaval. My small studio flat was becoming increasingly claustrophobic, and I was sure Skipper would appreciate a garden. After a long search, I had found the ideal one-bedroom flat with a garden, just round the corner.

I raided the supermarkets for cardboard boxes and began to cram my stuff into them. "Who would imagine you could get all this junk in this small flat!" exclaimed Ruth, who had come to help me pack. Skipper did not know what to make of packing. "Don't worry, you're going too, Skipper," Ruth assured him, carefully packing his toys in a small box. But he was not having that! He carefully unpacked the box, toy by toy.

I had to work the day before I was to move. We were doing a *Songs of Praise* from the West London Synagogue, and the first choir rehearsal was that day. As the programme was going to include a wide variety of Christian and Jewish music, Chris Mann asked me to go to the rehearsal. "You know everyone," he explained, "and some people may feel ill at ease in a synagogue, or might not remember that they have to wear cuppels (skullcaps). It would help if you could welcome everyone and see that they settle in." Skipper, I decided, would not get on with a cuppel, and he was in a funny mood because of our impending move.

"Could you look after Skipper for the afternoon and

evening?" I asked Olga, one of Skipper's favourite people.

"No problem," she replied. "Just bring him up to the *Heart-of-the-Matter* office before you go." I warned her that he was in a funny mood. "Don't worry," she reassured me, "he will get lots of walks and fuss."

I really enjoyed working on that Jewish-Christian *Songs of Praise*. The programme was about the work done by Christians and Jews in London towards understanding each other – celebrating their similarities and respecting their differences. The music was to reflect their common Old Testament heritage and show the way Christians had adapted the Jewish psalms. So it ranged ambitiously from a black Christian gospel choir version of a psalm to a traditional Catholic Gellineau psalm and we were going to have a go at singing in Hebrew as well.

It was the first time the black Christian choir had sung in a synagogue and wearing cuppels must have felt very strange to them. But they were willing to do so. "It is important that we show that we are all brothers, and can come together as such, and worship the same God," their minister told me. "We have suffered racial attacks in much the same way as the Jews have, and feel a certain solidarity with them. If we wear cuppels we only cover part of our heads and it is a compromise worth making to show what we have in common."

Rabbi Hugo Gryn welcomed everybody to the synagogue and demonstrated blowing the ram's horn, shofar. "I will blow the shofar to start the programme," he explained, "because it is always blown on special occasions such as New Year, and the fact that Christians and Jews of every denomination are coming together is a special occasion." As he blew it, an art which few acquire, I thought that the shofar must be one of the oldest musical instruments still in use, and remembered the damage it did to the walls of Jericho.

The shofar heralded a varied evening. Everybody had to learn everybody else's music in English and Hebrew. We began with the black Christian gospel version of Psalm 18, "I will call upon the Lord, for he is worthy to be

praised". Soon everybody had unwound and was singing rhythmically with the gospel choir. Next we had to
learn a Gellineau psalm. Our teacher was Felicity Elewes
from the Grail, a Roman Catholic organisation that aims
to use women in the church and had been instrumental
in translating Father Gellineau's French version of psalms
into English. "These psalms are set to old Hebrew chant
music," Felicity explained, "and it's very important to get
the emphasis and stress on the right words."

Everybody was also in for a long Hebrew lesson. As
the Christian hymn, "The God of Abraham Praise" is
based on a Hebrew doxology, we decided to sing it in
alternating verses of English and Hebrew. We were also
going to sing the Hebrew version of Psalm 133, "How
good and how pleasant it is for brothers to dwell together
in unity". Mercifully the synagogue had provided an
English-alphabet phonetic rendering of the Hebrew to
print in the *Songs of Praise* hymn books.

I was exhausted by the end of the rehearsal. But it
had been an exhilarating experience and I hoped it
would pave the way for more inter-faith programmes.
God can never be accused of making everybody the same,
so it is not surprising that we express our faith and
morality in a number of different religions. Who knows
who is right and who is wrong? I feel I have incorporated
ideas from many faiths into my own beliefs, which are
much richer as a result of this mingling of ideas.

"I've made so many new friends," a Christian lady
told me over the coffee and biscuits afterwards. "I've
actually been invited to a Sabbath meal next Friday!"

Everything was going so well and friendships were
being made as a result of the rehearsals. "That's a
bonus!" Chris Mann exclaimed, proudly packing away
the cuppel the synagogue had presented him with.

I had been so busy that I had not given Skipper much
thought – or the forthcoming move the next day! I went
round to Olga's to collect him, apologising for being so
late. Skipper was pleased to see me, but he was only wagging his tail at half-mast, something he does when he
knows he has been naughty. "Sit down and have a drink,"

Olga urged. "There's something I need to tell you." What had Skipper done? Olga was obviously not out of favour, because Skipper happily curled up on her knee and looked up at her as if to say, please don't tell tales.

"Don't worry, it's all right," Olga began. "It's just that Skipper has got a runny tummy. He must have been worried because you left him, and with all the packing at home, thought that you were moving without him."

"You poor little mite," I told Skipper, who dolefully wagged his tail at half-mast again, lapping up my sympathy.

"Now don't get upset; nobody's cross," Olga continued, "but Skipper had a little accident in Margery's office." Margery is the manager of Religious Programmes.

Skipper had never done anything like that before! I was appalled. "Don't worry," Olga reassured me. "Skipper is still Margery's friend and everyone was more worried about him than the cream-coloured carpet."

"Has he apologised to Margery?" I asked, remorseful and panic-stricken.

"He hasn't. You see, when I went down to clean up his mess, he slinked behind me and would not go near Margery's office. When I called him, he fled down the corridor and hid under David Kremer's desk."

I didn't know where to start apologising first: to Olga for having to clean up after him or Margery for her defiled cream carpet. I was near to tears.

*"Don't worry.* Everybody understands that he's upset about the move. We wouldn't be surprised if he was on the back streets of Stow-on-the-Wold because a family moved away and deserted him. Everybody is more worried about Skipper than the carpet. Promise."

The next morning I marched Skipper into the florist and supervised his purchase of a tasteful bunch of flowers. I then escorted him and his flowers to Margery's office. "He's come to apologise and he's brought you some flowers," I told her, dragging an embarrassed and resisting Skipper into the office.

"Thank you, Skipper. I'm not cross, really," Margery

assured him, and gave him a pat. The little eyes brightened and the tail slowly raised itself from half-mast for a sheepish wag. "Now go and move house, and forget about it," Margery told him.

I hoped that Skipper was going to be all right when we started moving. Nick and James were coming to help move us, so at least he wouldn't have strange men carrying off his things. I packed Skipper's toys, and put him in the box with them in an attempt to assure him that they and he were definitely coming. He suddenly sprang out of the box wagging his tail, as if to say, OK, now I know I'm coming! You're really not finishing with me!

He then decided to supervise the move. He followed Nick, James and me down the stairs with every load we packed in the van. He jumped in and out of it to ensure that everything was stowed carefully. Then he hopped into the driver's seat as we drove the two hundred yards down the road. When I unlocked the door, Skipper raced into his new flat and ran round and round, happily showing his approval. Then he hurtled out into the garden and christened it before happily pogoing around as we unloaded – his toys first. "All that fuss about nothing," I told him as he raced into the garden with his ball.

Nick and James were determined that Skipper should learn the new doorbell sound and where the phone was before they left. British Telecom had agreed to transfer my old phone to my new flat so that I would not have to wait until they ordered a new one. Suddenly Skipper charged against my knee and raced to the front-door. It was British Telecom come to fit my phone. "And there was I thinking we would have to ring the doorbell until he got the hang of the new sound," James commented. Skipper warily watched the stranger fit the phone and, as soon as it gave a trial ring, he enthusiastically answered it. I had never expected him to settle in so quickly after all the trauma he had gone through, but he showed his appreciation of his new flat by walking past the old one without even giving it a sniff on his way back from the park. If he had once had doubts about moving, they were definitely dispelled.

# 14

# Talk-Back

That inter-faith *Songs of Praise* from the West London Synagogue had been a high point for me. I knew it had been a good programme, but more importantly, it celebrated something that struck a responsive chord and meant a lot to me. Follow that, I thought, as I went back to work after moving flat. To my surprise I found I wasn't being asked to.

"There aren't any *Songs of Praise* for you to research until you go to Guernsey next month," Stephen explained, "so for the next four weeks you are to find house-hosts for *This is the Day*." *This is the Day* is a live morning-worship programme that comes from the home of a viewer every Sunday morning. The house-host participates in the programme by saying a little bit about themselves and then reads a lesson from one of the gospels and breaks a piece of bread as a sign of fellowship with the other viewers. "You'd better go and see David Craig, the producer, and find out what sort of people you have to look for," Stephen advised.

David was pleased to see me. "Our stock pile's running down," he explained ruefully. "We've been getting caught out recently, not having house-hosts lined up in the right places at the right time." What happens is that the *This is the Day* team suddenly get told there's going to be a mobile studio, called a scanner, somewhere between, say, Birmingham and Luton, and if they don't have a suitable name on their list, they have to find somebody in a hurry, and that's not easy. My brief was to find a supply of house-hosts from all over the country.

David proceeded to fill me in on what had to be taken into account. "For a start it's nice to be able to match the house-host with the theme for the week, but you'll find all sorts of less spiritual considerations coming first. Remember it's a live broadcast and not everyone can cope with that or feel at ease, praying with a television audience."

I wondered how I'd be able to assess this in advance.

"Another thing you must take into account is whether the house and the street are suitable. We bring three or four vans and there are two cameras in the room which need to be able to move around. And not everyone is happy to have a camera crew to stay for a weekend!"

I went away to have a think. The obvious place for me to start finding house-hosts was from all my good contacts on *Songs of Praise*. I soon had a long list, which was cut by over half when people were told the bit about it being a live broadcast. But quite a number still said they were interested and asked if I could come and discuss what was involved. "You're going on a long journey," I told Skipper in my best Gypsy Rose voice, as I mapped out a circular tour of the United Kingdom for us, and booked hire cars and hotels. "You'll probably be the best-travelled dog in the UK by the time the month's over." I packed my wellies beside a few weeks' supply of dog food in the car-boot.

"While you're on your travels, could you start by finding us a naval family in Plymouth to do a *This is the Day* in a month's time?" Stephen asked, giving me the addresses of the naval chaplains. That sounded fun, and I looked forward to Plymouth.

Most people didn't mind the inconvenience of the thirty film crew tramping through their house and their prize bits of furniture being shoved around, or even worse, removed from the house. What worried them was performing live. Remembering *Children in Need*, I knew how they felt and did my best to be re-assuring while explaining the essence of the pro-gramme. "Not everybody wants to see a church full of people on a Sunday morning. Maybe they have difficulty going to church themselves and feel alienated watching everybody worshipping together when they are house-bound. If we go to the house of a viewer who introduces him or herself, and invites everybody to worship, everybody is part of a live act of worship and this is what *This is the Day* is about. Everybody can participate in the programme by praying or breaking bread at home. And they can write in too, inviting people to pray for them or their friends or relatives in need."

Being deaf helped me to understand how someone can so easily become separated from a church or worshipping community. "I don't go to church now that I can't hear any more," one lady told me. "I don't know what is going on and when the service finishes, I have to talk to people, which is embarrassing."

"Why don't you go to one of the deaf churches?" I asked her.

"I don't want to. They are full of people like yourself who have always been deaf and they sign. I don't, and I'd feel even more disabled starting to learn to sign at my age."

The deaf are not the only disabled people who have problems joining a worshipping community. "We can't go to church because we can't take our dogs in and as braille hymn books are so massive, few churches have them," a blind couple once told me.

"I can't get my wheel-chair into a church and when the minister left, the new one didn't know about me, so until *This is the Day* came on, I had no way of worshipping," a lady in a wheel-chair confided. In fact, the more I research *Songs of Praise* and *This is the Day*, the more appalled I become. Elderly people, who find it difficult to go long distances because they have greater or lesser mobility problems, can no longer get to church, and at the time when they need its support the most. These are the people who are our regular *This is the Day* viewing fellowship.

I arrived in Plymouth to discover that I couldn't have timed things worse. It was the holiday period and most people were away. One of the few chaplains who was not on leave added a warning. "You're going to have problems, because most of the naval quarters are in small terrace houses in steep, narrow streets that won't be able to accommodate your vans and film crews." Nevertheless he had a list of people for me to see, all of whom would make first-rate house-hosts, but only one family could accommodate our vans, and even then it was a question of parking with the scanner van pointing down a hill.

"I'm sure the scanner can be propped up," Stephen reassured me. "However, I would like you to come to Plymouth when we do this programme to be on the floor and talk to the house-host and put the captions up at the right time."

I rapidly digested this. "Does that mean that I have to cope on talk-back?" I asked realising that I would have to understand what the director was saying in the scanner down the road if I was to put the captions up at the correct moment.

"Is that all right?" Stephen asked.

"No problem," I reassured him, trying to reassure myself.

Coping on talk-back was something that I knew I was going to have to do at some stage and I had given the matter a considerable amount of thought. I had reasoned that my subtitling amplifier could plug into a talk-back walkie-talkie. I went to Jackie and Jan, two of the production assistants. "Tell me all the sorts of things that get said on talk-back," I asked.

They were a little bewildered by my request, but complied. Most of it is pretty predictable: the production assistant counts down and calls the shots and the director makes comments, and in a live programme, might inform people of any sudden cuts. During the rehearsal the director will say to the camera man, "Can you get me a shot of this or that?" and the camera man will say whether he can or can't. Sometimes the director will ask someone to move something on the set or to tell the participants to do something.

Talk-back was predictable and there was a script for

the programme, but did I have the concentration to cope? I would not only have to keep an eye on what was being broadcast or filmed, I would also have to use every sense I possessed to cope with the talk-back at the same time. But I had two weeks to practise in.

I would watch television with subtitles, with my subtitling amplifier switched in to the television, and ask friends to talk to me at the same time. At first I hadn't got the concentration to do the two things at once and got tired quickly, but I persevered. Then I went to see an audiological engineer at Hearing Counsellors, the company that makes the ear-pieces the BBC use on talk-back, and explained that I wanted to connect my hearing-aid and subtitling amplifier to the talk-back system. I expected him to say that this was impossible but instead he said, "What a challenge."

"Think of a number of ways," I urged him, "just in case one doesn't work."

"I'll think of every conceivable way," he assured me.

All the same, I worried about things going wrong, about not coping, and putting the captions up at the wrong time. "Nothing is going to go wrong," I lectured myself. "Just keep calm."

The Friday that we were to drive down to Plymouth I went to collect my gadgets from Hearing Counsellors. "Our engineers and mould makers really enjoyed making these and are anxious to know how you get on, so do let us know, won't you?" they said. I thanked them and promised I would. My own determination would be useless without these people, I thought, remembering my battle to subtitle.

There was organised chaos in the *This is the Day* office. Everything that might be needed – Sellotape, Bibles, pieces of cardboard, staples, typewriters – was being packed into the boot of a hired car. When I had been a student I had had a glamorous view of television, and it did not include packing up cars with the contents of the entire office, but television is very down to earth.

After joining queues of weekend traffic on the roads out of London and on motorways we arrived very late.

But, by the time we reached Plymouth, I had memorised the script, so at least I could concentrate on hearing on talk-back, knowing what was being filmed at the same time. "I must *say* if I can't cope," I told myself, but somehow I knew that things were going to be all right.

The Bentleys – Sandra, our house-host and her husband Paul – were pleased to see us on Saturday morning and while their children were given a tour of the vans by the technical crew, the rest of us set about making their living-room unrecognisable. "If you're unhappy about anything, please say," I urged them as Roger decided to move a picture, so that it was in the middle of the set.

"I'll get a hammer and a nail," Paul happily volunteered.

"Do you want coffee?" Sandra asked.

"Yes, but I'll make it," I volunteered, "and we've brought our own paper cups, coffee and milk."

"You shouldn't have," Sandra replied, shocked. "But you must all have lunch. How many will there be?"

After I'd made an ocean of coffees, I sneaked away to try out my talk-back. I got out my screwdriver and attached system one. Would I hear anything? Please God, let me hear something! I prayed as I turned it on. I did hear something, but it was very, very far away. I turned up the volume, and to my delight I could hear something that was loud but distorted! Wonderful, I thought, I can work on this.

"I hate to tell you, but it's so loud we can all hear what's going on," Jeff, the stage manager, told me ruefully. "You'll have to stop the volume spilling somehow or we'll be broadcasting your talk-back as well." I went away and began to make some adjustments. If I was in the scanner and directing, I wouldn't have this problem, I thought. It's only because I'm in the room where we're broadcasting from. I tightened up the connection between my amplifier and my hearing-aid, sure that that was where the spillage was coming from. "Is this all right?" I asked.

Jeff listened carefully. "Yes, that's fine now, but don't

worry, we'll soon tell you if we can hear it!" I was relieved, but I still had a long way to go.

I could hear the sound, but it was muddled. I made an effort to pull myself together and concentrate, when Roger, the director, walked into the room. "I've been trying to call you for the last twenty minutes," he said with discernible restraint.

"Oh, I wasn't operational then, but I am now," I told him.

"Well, we're going to do the letters when the letter readers arrive, but until then we'll do some filming around the house to supplement the film that we've brought with us." With that he went.

The letter readers, who were to read viewers' letters for us, were mostly friends and colleagues of the Bentley family and could hardly recognise the house. I crammed them into the children's bedroom with John Whale, who was going to produce the letters. "All the letter readers are here," I informed Roger on talk-back, and concentrated, waiting for his reply.

"All right, I'll record the letters in ten minutes," he replied. I got most of that. I could also gather that Roger was recording a street scene outside by looking at the monitor and supplementing that with the talk-back. It was like subtitling all over again. I hoped I could keep up this concentration for the rest of the day. I was not hearing everything – an odd phrase came through the jumble of sound. "OK, we'll do the letters now," came through the talk-back. Before anyone could accuse me of not responding I informed the readers, nervously waiting, that their hour had arrived.

I spent the rest of the morning getting what I could from the talk-back, feeling relieved that I had had the sense to ask Jackie and Jan what kind of things were said on it. "Move that vase," I heard Roger say as we were about to record Paul doing a reading. I quickly moved the vase. "Tell Paul to wear his jumper; it looks better." I only heard Paul and jumper, but guessed the rest and handed it to him.

My confidence was gradually increasing, but the worst

was still to come, I reminded myself. During the Saturday morning, we were only recording the "wallpaper" film: letters and readings. That afternoon and evening we would have a full run-through and then I would have to put up the dreaded captions. I felt really sick. "I can't do this," I began to gibber.

Just then Sandra, who knew it was my first time on talk-back, came up to me. "If you can manage during a live-broadcast, then so can I," she said. I remembered that I was supposed to be giving Sandra confidence, not the other way round, and stopped worrying about my own problems.

"Now you've got going, you are managing very well," said Roger at lunch-time, "and you're keeping everyone calm and happy." This encouraged me.

"And you're not deafening us with your talk-back now," laughed Jeff.

"Don't worry about when to break the bread, or light the candle," I assured Sandra. "We show you a board with the order things are to happen on it, and Jeff will tell you what to do when."

"Gosh!" said Sandra, relieved. "I thought I'd have to remember everything."

I sorted the captions out and put the appropriate ones beside the right cameras. "You do camera A and I'll do camera B," Jeff suggested. As the living-room was small, we knelt down on the floor, out of the way of the camera. "I hope you move quickly," Jeff warned, "because you've only got a minute to change caption F to caption G."

"No problem," I assured him. Keep calm, I told myself, pray, concentrate and have confidence, and all will be well.

I heard Jackie, the production assistant, calling the shots. I could see the programme on the monitor. I heard Roger saying, "That's not quite right, we'll have to do that again," or "That looks blank, what can we put there?" Everything was predictable – sensible, possible and likely. All the same, I was shaking when I moved the first caption and replaced it with the next one as the appropriate shot was called.

"Tilt it a bit towards the camera," I heard Roger say, then, "A bit further back." Nice and predictable. Sometimes I didn't decipher the mess of words, but I kept calm. Sandra also kept calm, with Paul anxiously watching.

"I never thought that there was so much to breaking bread or lighting candles," she joked as we rehearsed her timing on these.

"Light the candle just as the gospel fanfare starts," the stage manager told her. "Watch me and I'll cue you."

As soon as the rehearsals were over, I felt like collapsing in a heap. My ear ached and I was shattered with having to concentrate so much, but delighted to have succeeded in doing everything right. I thanked Jeff and the camera man for being so patient with me. "That's what we're here for," they told me, "and it made it more worthwhile for us."

I also congratulated Sandra, who had been a perfect house-host. "I only hope I stay as calm tomorrow," she laughed.

Anything could still go wrong, but I knew it wouldn't. If I ever doubted the power of the Almighty, I didn't then, because I knew that everything would be fine, just like Sandra did. Throughout my sleepless night, I never expected to be so strong and confident, but I was unnaturally so the next morning as we assembled at seven a.m. in Paul and Sandra's church hall, where members of their church had volunteered to do a breakfast for the crew.

The final rehearsal went all right, but as we were running too long, we cut some captions out of the programme. Before we went on the air I checked with the stage manager, to make sure that I correctly understood all the changes, just to be on the safe side. Paul came and stood behind me. "I don't know whether to watch or not," he confided, feeling for Sandra. He eventually decided to watch.

I was shaking when I heard, "Stand by" and "On air", and I remember waiting with trepidation for the first caption, making sure that I was not in the camera's way. We must have looked ridiculous, crawling all over the floor, arranging newspapers or captions, then scooping them up and dashing out of the way before the camera picked us up or ran us over. I was listening intently for the shots in case Roger made any changes to the running order whilst we were on air. The half an hour seemed like hours, but it was soon over and I hoped I had not done anything wrong. I hadn't, and neither had Sandra, although she had had a nervous moment when the first match broke as she was lighting the candle.

Afterwards there was coffee and congratulations amid the furniture rearranging, and all the time I had this feeling of exhilaration at having met and overcome one more challenge. I could use talk-back. During the programme a letter asking people to pray for hearing-impaired people had been read. Had this been coincidence? I wondered. Something had certainly helped me that day.

I had left Skipper with my parents for the Plymouth weekend, and as soon as I returned I went to collect him. "Well done," said dad. "We both watched the programme with our hearts in our mouths, but nothing went wrong."

"Really?" I asked. "The captions didn't wobble, or come up at the wrong time?"

"No," mum firmly assured me, "we'd have told you if something did go wrong." I relaxed. I knew that they would be honest with me.

"However, we are very pleased that you've come for Skipper."

"Why? Has he been naughty?" I asked, remembering cream carpets.

"Well," mum began, "he won't tell us when the phone or the doorbell go, and he usually does when you're away. This time he just lies there as if to say, aren't you going to answer that?"

"I hope we haven't done something to put him off his stroke," added dad.

147

So mum hurried to the phone and asked a family friend to ring to put Skipper through his paces now that I had returned. All was well. As soon as the phone rang, he came and fetched me. We then tried the doorbell, and he did not fail me then, either. "Maybe he's got used now to working in a large office and only having to respond for me," I suggested.

"I know what it was," said mum perceptively, "he thought that he was on holiday here, and while you were away he wasn't going to do any work for two people he knew didn't need it!"

I had been worried about coping in Plymouth and mum and dad had been out of their minds worrying about Skipper forgetting his skills. Meanwhile Skipper had been enjoying a well-earned holiday. I was glad one of us had had a relaxing weekend.

## 15

# Islands of the Spirit

Travelling is something that is in my blood. My Iranian ancestors came from a tribal background, as did my Irish ones – the O'Byrnes were one of the last wandering tribes of Ireland. Even my grandmother's maiden name was Chapman! After I graduated and started work, I began to put aside some money so I could travel. I was fascinated by the idea of meeting people of different countries, cultures and faiths and ventured to Israel, Russia and North India. By the time I started work on *Songs of Praise* the idea of travelling long distances and being away for long periods of time did not bother me. However, when I was due to research a *Songs of Praise* from the Bailliwick of Guernsey, I did become very worried, not at the idea of travelling, but about taking Skipper on a plane. Gillian at Hearing Dogs assured me that it would be all right for Skipper to travel by plane, but Channel flights risked being diverted to France if the weather was unreliable, and that would mean an automatic six-month quarantine for Skipper on his return to Britain. I couldn't face that gamble and didn't have the time to go by boat as I was due in Sidmouth the next week, so I went to Guernsey alone and Skipper had a holiday with Gillian and Gemma.

One day they took him along to a local show in the New Forest where Hearing Dogs had an information stall. Being small, they plonked him on the counter where people made a fuss of him all the afternoon and he spent a lot of time blissfully rolling on his back, waving his paws in the air. Gillian was selling copies of a children's story about a Hearing Dog called Buttons, who looked remarkably like Skipper. This was not entire coincidence. Sir Hugh Casson, who had illustrated the book, had borrowed some photos of Hearing Dogs and it was clearly Skipper's photo that had inspired him. So, children were coming up saying, "Oh, look, there's Buttons!" and asking for his autograph. Never one to disappoint his public over a small matter like a signing session, Skipper was taken off to get his paws muddy and spent the rest of the afternoon shamelessly autographing a book he had never written a word of.

Meanwhile, I was finding Guernsey fascinating. Going over to the tiny off-shore island of Herm on the mid-day ferry was like stepping back in time. Its simplicity of lifestyle reminded me of the tranquillity I had found on my travels in Asia.

"It's so peaceful and quiet here," I said to Major Peter Wood, who has been tenant of Herm since 1947.

"Surely everywhere is quiet when one is deaf?" one of his family asked, genuinely puzzled.

I tried to explain what I meant. "When I was walking in the Galilean hills and in the hills in Srinagar and Ladakh, there was an empty silence – a vacuum. There was no hassle of everyday life – and something just opened up, and a feeling of peace came over me. Herm has this same feeling."

In our busy lives we tend to forget simple things that are very important as we rush around doing this and that; I remember sitting round a camp fire when we were stuck in a landslide on the endless mountain journey from Srinagar in Kashmir to Ladakh. We could not get much food as we were miles from anywhere, so the lorry drivers and my fellow travellers had pooled what food, booze and cigarettes they could muster. The booze and cigarettes proved to be revolting, illegal home-made versions, stiff with questionable substances.

The Indians were interested to know where we came from, and how we lived and we were just as interested in them, and many a laborious, interpreted conversation took place around the camp fires. One Indian told me that he was a farmer on a pilgrimage to a monastery, where a great lama from Sikkim was due to visit. It was important that he was a farmer, he told me, because his children could see what their father did and follow him when he passed on. They knew that he tended their small field, looked after their few animals and birds and fought the endless drought. His work was their survival. They could also see their mother run the home and carry the family's wealth on her headdress in turquoises. It took me a long time to explain city life to him and the role of a working mother, but when I did, many of the Indians were surprised. "If father and mother are not there, is there really a family? How do children understand that their parents provide for them?"

Major Wood smiled when he heard this story. "That was one of the reasons we came to Herm. Like your Indian farmer, we felt it important that the traditional family roles were kept. On Herm the children know that I am responsible for, say, the generator, and that so-and-so's dad is responsible for milking the cows. They understand what their parents do and respect that."

Later that evening on Herm, when I sat overlooking Bear's Bay, Skipperless, with only my thoughts for company, I remembered more roadside conversations on the way to Ladakh. "Many people in the West think that we are poor," one jovial Indian remarked. "But we are more rich than the sahibs. Why? True, there isn't always enough to eat or there may be no doctor when we need one. But we have our family and friends and we are rich. Sahibs have freezers, fridges, cameras and pop music, which I would like, but they forget how good people are."

A young man, who had studied in Oxford on an Indian government grant, was interpreting for me, and he added his own observations. "I see much material love in the West. Parents show love for their children by buying them things, but I never saw a sister carry her younger sister or brother, or a parent going without a meal for his child." I assured him that some Westerners do go without for their children in many different ways, but wondered just how much the West has forgotten the simple, important things these men were speaking about.

When we eventually reached Leh, the capital of Ladakh, I climbed the rocky hill that led to a solitary Buddhist monastery overlooking the city. Just above the monastery is the palace, a model of the Potala at Lhasa in Tibet. It was daybreak, and the sun was just beginning to lift its scorching rays over the sandy, table-topped plateau that Leh was seated on.

"There's a dog barking!" warned Mary, my companion. We looked up, and high above our heads, an angry-looking dog was leaning out of the monastery window, having a good bark. "It's a Lhasa Apso," I said, delighted, "like Miss Lion in the Spiderman comics. They're sometimes called Careful Lion Dogs and they are the guardians of Tibetan temples."

"Well, it was him and his fellow guardians that kept me awake last night," Mary sighed. "You know, you are lucky not to hear at times. You must have been the only person who slept last night."

The dogs had alerted the monks to our arrival and they proudly invited us into the temple. We reverently took off our shoes and walked over the floor tacky with rancid yak butter. In front of us, at the far end of the temple, were peaceful Buddhas, but behind us, on either side of the door, were angry Tantric deities, whose fierce, primitive presence tests the depth of one's meditation, dispelling spiritual pride. Gazing on the serenity of the Buddha, may make you think that you have gained the mental and spiritual peace of nirvana. But a departing glance at the Tantric demons can shatter this illusion. Only when you reach a genuine state of nirvana can the demons hold no terrors.

I respect the way that Buddhism and Hinduism are ways of life as much as beliefs. The people struggle to live the way of the dharma, the way of life. By doing this, they hope that the pāpa (evil) will not taint their souls and spoil their chances of a better reincarnation and eventual release into nirvana from the round of reincarnations. Many live out the dharma in spirit and action. We in the West often treat our Christianity as a piece of weekly routine that comes between the Sunday papers and the Sunday roast, and we are too busy thinking of other things to meditate on what our religion should mean to us. We are certainly not prepared or even required to give up things for our faith.

When I visited Russia, I escaped from the official tour of endless Moscow war memorials and industrial achievements to meet a Soviet dissident that a journalistic colleague had befriended. To meet her I travelled to the end of the Moscow underground. The sight was depressing. There were skyscrapers, standing one behind the other in a wasteland. It was a cold winter's day and children had made fires on the bare earth around the grey skyscrapers. Instantly Eliot's words flooded into my mind:

I will show you something different
from either your shadow at morning standing
    behind you,
or your shadow at evening striding to meet you –
I will show you fear in a handful of dust.

"I am taking you to my home," my Russian friend told me. "I want you to see it and to tell others what you see. I would like to give you lunch, so we will go shopping on the way home." We joined a long queue outside a shop. When we at last saw the food counter there was a chicken and a few mangy sausages for sale. The champagne and cakes were more abundant, and cheaper. Armed with a bottle of champagne and a heavy cake, we entered one of the monstrous blocks. The lifts were not working, and the banister wobbled dangerously. The grey regulation paint was faded and peeling.

Eventually we reached my friend's home. The inside reminded me of student flats, though my hostess was well past that stage of her career. Fading ballet posters weighed down the drooping yellow wallpaper. These were soon joined by some Torvill and Dean pictures I had brought. "I love Torvill and Dean," she told me. "Everything about them is free. However good Russian skaters and dancers are, they will never dance with freedom because they don't know it." She then explained how she had had a good job and a lovely flat in central Moscow, until it was discovered that she was a Christian and interested in meeting Westerners. She was then forced to move to her present flat and lost her job and privileges. "In a way I am now free," she told me. "My neighbours will report that I listen to the World Service and that you came, but they know because I no longer make a secret of it. I am silenced, but in my silence, I have become free."

The evening on Herm was a wonderful opportunity to think about my travels and the people I had encountered, but the next day it was back to the hurly-burly of researching the programme. I felt sad to say goodbye to the hospitable Wood family as I joined the milk churns on the milk ferry to Guernsey. I had a whole list of people to visit on Guernsey, and finding my way was no joke. The map of the island was excellent, but many lanes and houses were unmarked.

I met the De La Salle brothers, a Roman Catholic teaching order responsible for the well-known tourist attraction, the Little Chapel, still being decorated within and without with thousands of pieces of broken china and glass, set in the plaster walls. Smashing china is an art, the brothers assured me. A Pope Paul souvenir mug was lovingly smashed in demonstration, and the papal face beamed intact from the pieces. I wanted a go. Reluctantly the monks offered me an old plate and told me to break it into four pieces. Smithereens – they were right!

I also met an amazing artist who had painted Noah's animals queuing up to go into a space rocket. They were depicted waiting on Bear's Beach on Herm, where the arrival of such a craft would have created quite a sensation. Looking at the painting, I was left in no doubt that nuclear holocaust was the twentieth century equivalent to the biblical flood. The artist's wife was a school-teacher and she pointed me on my way to the next port of call. "He's one of my pupils. I'll draw you a map and describe the house."

Edward was a young man of thirteen with spina bifida. His mother had been interviewed on *Songs of Praise* when it came to Guernsey seven years ago, and we were all anxious to know how he was getting on. Famously was the answer! "I'm in training for the Milk Run half-marathon," Edward told me excitedly. "The Disabled Sports Association have lent me a special wheel-chair to do it in, and every evening I go round the lanes in it to get fit."

Edward was going to be the first person in a wheelchair to attempt the Guernsey half-marathon, and he hoped to raise money for the Disabled Sports Association and the Christian Union at his school. Luckily we had our film crew the weekend of the race, so we were able to film Edward starting off an hour early. "I don't want to finish last," he confided to our viewers. He need not have worried, he finished with a better time than he had anticipated and the look on his face as he crossed the line said it all.

It was decided to interview Edward in the church during the recording of the hymns – quite an ordeal for anybody, but Edward was undaunted. "Do you ever take that medal off?" Ian Gall, our presenter, asked.

"Only to go to bed!" replied Edward, casting yet another glance at it.

Later, Ian confided that it was the most moving moment of his *Songs of Praise* career when he asked Edward the next question. "Why have you chosen the hymn, 'My Life Is Really Blessed'?"

Edward paused and looked down at his legs, rendered useless because of a hole in his spine, and then replied, "Because I feel that my life is blessed, even though I am what I am."

# 16

# I Climb a Silent Wall

It had been a hectic summer, we had travelled all over the UK and at times Skipper and I began to wonder where we lived and what town we were in. During this time I saw very little of my parents, and away from home and my special phones that allowed me to talk to family and friends, I sometimes felt very lonely and isolated. But Skipper was marvellous company. He has great resilience and is a natural traveller, hopping as nonchalantly into hired cars as any business tycoon, making himself at home in every hotel. Each new town is "his" town within hours of his arrival as he finds new haunts and walks. But every time we return home for a day or night, he is pleased to be back, and wastes no time in inspecting his garden.

Once, on our way to Worcester, we chanced to pass the National Canine Defence League kennels at Evesham, where Skipper was discovered by Tony and recruited for Hearing Dogs. I couldn't resist a visit. The kennels were very welcoming, especially as Skipper was now a famous son, with a newspaper cutting about us pinned up in the office. I was shown the kennels where the dogs go when they first come to the NCDL. Sometimes their owners claim them, but if they are not claimed after a week, they go into some other kennels. Skipper had only been in a couple of days when Tony discovered him, so he had to wait and see if he was going to be claimed. Nobody did then and nobody has since his furry face and his Stow-on-the-Wold origins have been broadcast in the media. All of which leads one to the conclusion that he wasn't so much lost as abandoned. Most dogs are abandoned, the manager admitted. "People will just drive to this area and let them out of the car and callously drive away. Some even do this on the M5. The police then hand them in to us, unless the dog is run over first." I felt sad and sick. How can we British call ourselves animal lovers? I thought. In the office we checked up on Skipper's documentation. I had his vaccination certificate on me with his number, L128, so it was not long before we found the appropriate entry. "L128 – Terrier, white, black and tan. Male – Stow-on-the-Wold."

"The Stow police would have brought him to us," the manager explained. "He could have run off, maybe, from a gypsy camp. There are quite a few in the area." I sighed; it looked like Skipper's past would remain a mystery.

"What date did he arrive?" I asked, determined to learn the last shred of detail.

The manager consulted his records again. "He was handed in on the 27th June 1984," he told me. "But that's my birthday!" I exclaimed. No wonder Skipper and I were made for each other.

That summer was hard work and demanded enormous concentration. As well as lonely, I often felt drained at the end of a day, but it is a job I love doing, and you know it's worthwhile when somebody you are interviewing pours out their story of suffering and hardship saying, "I don't really want to be interviewed on your programme, but if you think hearing what happened to me and how I coped will help other people in a similar situation, well, all right, I'm willing to do it." That is one thing television is good at: helping people to share their problems and draw strength and comfort from others. I know I myself learn day by day from the people I meet in connection with *Songs of Praise.* Their experiences give me strength and help me to continue to come to terms with my own problem and to learn that really, I am not so badly off.

I never forget the day I was to see a young man in his

thirties suffering from multiple sclerosis. He had lost everything from his job downwards as he gradually succumbed to the disease. I was determined to arrive on time as I did not want to keep him waiting. When I drove up I found the door already open for me on a cold winter's night. The young man was waiting by it. "I opened the door for you because they told me that you were deaf," he began, consciously making his slurred speech clearer with a great effort. "I was worried that you would come, ring the bell and if I took a long time to answer it, think I wasn't in and go. I have an answerphone, you see, and I reassure whoever is waiting that I am coming to open the door, but I thought you wouldn't hear it."

I tried to choke back tears. Countless times I had told people that I was deaf and couldn't cope with an answerphone, yet encountered them all the same and had to put my hand on the loudspeaker to feel it vibrate and more often than not got in a muddle with them, to my embarrassment. But here was this young man with so many worsening problems of his own who had been so incredibly thoughtful on behalf of someone else's disability.

I arrived back from a trip to Dumfries to find a huge package on my desk. I wondered what on earth could be inside, and opened it hastily to discover a Vistel Mark 2. I couldn't believe it! For the past few months I had been asking Religious Programmes for a Vistel like the one in Ceefax.

There was a note on the machine saying a Vistel Mark 1 was also on the way. You need two, one at each end, for a conversation. The Mark 2 is bulky and can't be used in phone boxes, but it can store messages. The Mark 1 is typewriter-size and portable, and the two couplets can be connected to an ordinary telephone handset. It has a small visual display just above the keys and you can have a typewritten conversation with the other Vistel. It's a boon to me when I get stuck somewhere on location, maybe the hire car hasn't turned up, and I need to get through to the office. I was thrilled.

There was another surprise: a BBC envelope on my desk which looked important. I remembered I had applied for an assistant producer's job in the department, which I knew I was not qualified for, but I was due to leave Religious Programmes in September. This would be a rejection. I braced myself to open the envelope. But it was not a rejection letter at all. It was offering me a permanent researcher's post in Religious Programmes. I had hoped at best for another six-month extension, but never a permanent job. I scooped up the unsuspecting Skipper and hugged him. "I bet they only wanted to keep you," I told him.

"Not true!" cried everybody.

There is no way that I can say exactly what getting a permanent job in a part of the BBC that isn't connected with the deaf meant to me. I suppose that most of all it confirmed that I was a person, who just happens to be deaf; that nobody has given me the job because they felt sorry for me – I had competed and won it fair and square. The only allowances that are made for me are having Skipper in the office and my special telephones and equipment. And I am thankful that my ability to do a job is judged on my performance with Skipper and these telephones, not without them.

"We're all going on a works outing to Windsor, do you want to come?" It was a day of surprises. I eagerly said yes, but nearer the time worried about whether or not I should take Skipper and whether perhaps the others would want to go somewhere he wouldn't be allowed. It was too hot for leaving him in a car. In the end I tried to chicken out on the day. But nobody would hear of it! "You and Skipper are coming, and that's an order," said Stephen.

"You're both coming with me and Clare in my car," Chris Mann announced, "and in case you start on the 'Skipper won't be allowed anywhere nonsense', the definition of where we're going is where Skipper is allowed. The outing won't be the same without him, so come on."

We all met at Windsor station, Roger Royle clutching

a massive BBC2 umbrella to make sure it wouldn't rain. Skipper enjoyed being rowed up the river and sat importantly on a cushion looking out for a good picnic spot for us. He then managed to persuade the man on a hamburger stand to donate three over-cooked hamburgers to the Starving Hearing Dogs Fund. After lunch we all decided to play rounders with Skipper's ball. I rather fancied my batting, as I'd been in the Battle Abbey rounders team. But I'd reckoned without the big hitting of Roger Royle, an expertise gained no doubt from his days as a chaplain at Eton. Skipper was no support to me at all. Full of hamburger, he went to sleep under a tree.

"This outing wouldn't have been the same without Skipper," Jan commented as we walked back to the cars. I said that I was sure that that was not the case. "Oh, yes!" Jan insisted. "Skipper has made us all much more . . . human in a way. He's brought us all so much happiness. He's as much a part of the team as you are." Jan's words meant so much and reminded me of so much – that if it was not for the team of my family, friends, teachers and colleagues and Skipper, I would not have had the strength and courage to climb a silent wall and land on the other side.